Introduction

In many ways, pregnancy and birth are the perfect preparation for parenting.

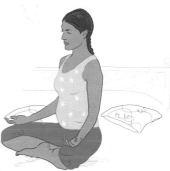

Like birth, parenting can be unpredictable; it forces us to move beyond our comfort zone and challenges us to constantly grow. Becoming a parent takes courage. It's a sometimes scary, often surprising, deeply moving and profoundly rewarding experience, and pregnancy is just the beginning of that journey.

During labour, there often comes a point when the woman is convinced she can't go on – it's almost as if she hits a wall, and has absolutely no idea how to continue. What amazes me every time is watching her discover deep within herself a strength she didn't know she had, and find a way to keep going. This is how childbirth transforms us: it pushes us beyond our known capacities, and teaches us something remarkable about ourselves.

I've written this book with this in mind. What you have in your hand is an introduction to the start of your journey, but much of the knowledge you will draw upon along the way is already within you. I will cover the basic biological changes during pregnancy, important nutrition and health recommendations, and many natural remedies for the numerous aches and pains of pregnancy. I'll equip you with information to help you make decisions about the location of your birth, your healthcare provider and your labour support team, and offer plenty of tips for the postnatal period and newborn care.

But remember that this is just the beginning. Every pregnant woman's journey is different, and it is my hope that this book helps you to start charting your own personal course and that you find empowerment in every step along the way.

Ali Monaghan

① Am I really pregnant?

Your period may be a few days late, your breasts may be unusually tender. Perhaps you've had a strange feeling which you can't seem to shake. However you first suspect that you're pregnant, confirmation of it marks the beginning of a transformative journey.

Signposts to pregnancy

One of the very first signs of pregnancy, and usually the most obvious, is a missed period. If you have irregular cycles or a very busy life, it may take a few weeks before you realize that your period hasn't arrived. In contrast, if your cycle is like clockwork or you've been tracking it very carefully, sometimes being even a single day late is enough to confirm your growing suspicions.

Changes in your breasts can also clue you in to the fact that you're pregnant. These changes are similar to the premenstrual changes which you may normally experience, but are usually a bit stronger and more intense. Your breasts can feel swollen and full, and can sometimes be extra-sensitive and tender to the touch, even painfully so. You may also experience a tingling sensation and the nipples can become hypersensitive – this is when a more supportive bra can really come in handy! Fortunately, the uncomfortable feelings usually resolve by the end of the first trimester, although your breasts will continue to grow and change throughout the pregnancy (read more about this on page 28).

Other early pregnancy signs include fatigue, nausea, vomiting, appetite changes and frequent urination – we'll focus on these changes and how to cope with them in the next chapter. Eventually, the time will come to confirm your suspicions with hard evidence. This is usually done by breaking out the trusty home pregnancy test, which checks your urine for the presence of a hormone known as human chorionic gonadotropin, or hCG. Remarkably, these small and ubiquitous urine dipsticks can be up to 99 per cent accurate. However, if the test is taken too early, it can give a false negative (it says you're not pregnant when you are), and there are a few drugs and medicines that can sometimes cause a false positive result (indicating that you are pregnant when you're not). If you had a negative result but you still don't have your period, wait a week then test again. Your midwife or doctor may also confirm your pregnancy through a pelvic examination.

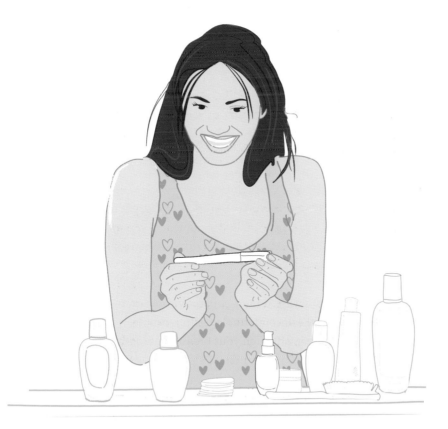

Of course, the most definitive confirmation of pregnancy is either an early ultrasound scan that clearly shows a growing embryo with a positive foetal heart beat, or a blood test showing rising serum levels of hCG, which are 99 per cent accurate (in the case of the ultrasound, 100 per cent accurate). However, these tests are usually reserved for women who are experiencing symptoms that warrant further investigation, such as bleeding or spotting, or for women who are undergoing infertility treatments. The majority of pregnancies can be confirmed by a missed period and a positive urine pregnancy test alone.

How far along am I?

Conventional wisdom holds that a pregnancy is nine months long, but the medical profession defines a pregnancy as lasting 40 weeks, or 280 days. This is because they begin the count from the start of your last menstrual period; that's approximately two weeks before sperm even met egg. And they divide the pregnancy into three trimesters, or three-month periods. You'll definitely want to keep track, so here are a few tips to help you make sense of the dating:

• Think about your pregnancy in terms of weeks, rather than months. In these terms, 4 weeks is when you miss your period, 20 weeks is halfway through and 40 weeks is your due date.
• Look up your due date on the calendar and note what day of the week it falls on; then, every week, when you hit that same day, you can add another week to your count.
• Babies rarely arrive exactly on their due date. Any point after 37 weeks is considered full term, so plan to have everything prepared at least three weeks before your official due date.

The good news

For a lot of women, the positive result on the urine dipstick brings feelings of giddiness, excitement and happy anticipation. Pregnancy may have been something you've been looking forward to for years, and now that it has actually happened, it's thrilling to begin to think about the changes that are on their way.

> Three days late. Time to break out the bottle of...sparkling apple juice? #fingerscrossed

It's fun to walk around with the secret for a while, knowing that there's something special going on which you're carrying with you everywhere you go, invisible to the world but known to you. Many women ride out their pregnancy on rolling waves of peace and contentment.

Or not so great...

However, statistics suggest that around 80 per cent of women feel less than ecstatic about the news. Their feelings might include disappointment, anxiety or unhappiness when they first find out they're pregnant. Pregnancy marks the beginning of an irreversible and life-changing journey, so it's very understandable to want to take a step back into a pre-pregnant life. It can also be difficult to talk about these feelings, because the general expectation is to view the pregnancy as a purely joyful or positive event. Acknowledging negative or ambivalent feelings may seem like an admission of failure or inadequacy, and trigger a self-administered guilt trip: 'If I were a good mother, I'd be happy about this'. The truth is, good mothers aren't always happy. They're human.

Condensed idea
It takes a while to believe that you really are pregnant

② A changing body

While your body will soon start to undergo radical changes, hardly any of them are visible at the start of the pregnancy. But you'll notice some changes, such as the way you'll feel more tired, less like eating and possibly nauseous. This isn't great, but it is normal.

Morning sickness

There are women who sail through pregnancy feeling fabulous the entire time, and if you are one of these lucky women, enjoy! For the majority of women, however, the first trimester involves some combination of nausea, vomiting and fatigue. In fact, up to 70 per cent of all women report symptoms of morning sickness. The good news is that for most women it is short-lived, lasting from weeks 5–8 of the pregnancy to around 13–16 weeks.

> Nauseous, tired, and is it just me or are my jeans already hard to do up?? #andsoitbegins

We still don't fully understand the cause; certainly the higher hormone levels of pregnancy have something to do with it, but other theories have suggested that low blood sugar, slowed digestion, the growing uterus and emotional changes may play a role. You might also be wondering why it's called morning sickness, as it can happen at any point during the day.

Unfortunately, there's no easy cure, but the text box opposite offers some tried-and-tested suggestions that might help. Experiment with different things, and stick to what works for you. If you do find yourself vomiting, make sure you remain well hydrated; water, sports drinks (most of which include rehydration salts), coconut water or bouillon (a kind of thin broth) can all help replenish lost electrolytes and rehydrate you. Unfortunately, vomiting anywhere from 4 to 8 times in a day can be normal during the first trimester, but if you find yourself vomiting more than eight times in one day or feel like you can't keep anything down, check with your midwife or doctor and ask them what the next step is.

Natural remedies

Alternative medicine can also come to your aid. Studies have shown that acupressure, especially on the Pericardium 6 (P6) point, can steady the vomiting reflex. If you're feeling nauseous, try locating the P6 spot: it's about 3 cm (1 in) up from your wrist, between the two tendons on the inside of your arm; the correct spot will feel strangely painful. Gently

Stomach soothers

Work your way down this list of comfort measures for morning sickness, and go with whatever works best for you.

- Eat small and frequent snacks every 2–3 hours.
- Avoid greasy or fatty foods.
- Avoid anything which doesn't smell appealing to you or makes you feel queasy.
- Keep some dry crackers beside your bed at night and eat one or two in the morning before getting up.
- Choose foods that are high in protein rather than high in carbohydrate.
- Drink ginger, peppermint or camomile tea.
- Drink a glass of low-acidic juice before going to bed (such as papaya, pear, peach or apricot).

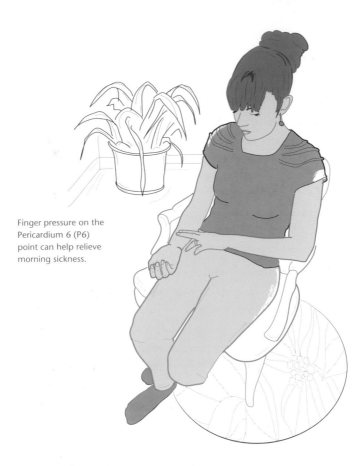

Finger pressure on the Pericardium 6 (P6) point can help relieve morning sickness.

massage that point and the nausea should subside. You can purchase wristbands that apply continuous pressure from health food stores and pharmacies. Acupuncture has also been used to treat morning sickness with great success (read more on page 86).

Vitamin B6 has been found to help with morning sickness. However, the medical profession is still researching the safety of taking large doses of any vitamin during pregnancy, so if you want to try increasing your intake of B6, take a prenatal multivitamin supplement or eat more foods that are rich in the vitamin (such as chicken, tuna, salmon or apricots). If none of these remedies work, ask your doctor's advice. Anti-nausea medication is always an option, but this is usually reserved as a last resort.

Not hungry?

Unsurprisingly, you may feel like you have little to no appetite in the first trimester, often because everything is making you nauseous. If this happens, try to eat at least something (a piece of fruit, dry toast, a muesli bar or some yogurt) every 2–3 hours, and keep yourself hydrated. Sometimes a smoothie will stay down more easily than actual food. If you find yourself losing a few pounds during the first trimester, this can be normal as well. Most women find their appetites waiting for them again shortly after they enter the second trimester.

Get more sleep!

One of the other common signs of early pregnancy is fatigue – with a capital F. The cause seems obvious – in addition to everything else you're doing in your busy day, your body is also hard at work creating an entire human being from scratch. You might need several naps throughout the day, a 9 p.m. bedtime, or weekend mornings devoted to sleeping in until your body naturally wakes up on its own. These early weeks of pregnancy are crucial times of development for your baby, so try to prioritize your rest as much as you can.

Even though you're exhausted, you might also find yourself getting up to go to the bathroom more often. Frequent urination is common at the start and the end of the pregnancy. In the beginning, the growing uterus applies a great deal of pressure to your bladder, giving it very little room in which to expand and making it feel as if you have to pee every hour or so. Thankfully, once the uterus grows out of the pelvis and begins to enter the abdomen, this feeling eases for a few months.

Condensed idea
Morning sickness can be miserable, but it's usually short-lived

(3) Changing relationships

Your mind is probably abuzz with all the changes under way – in your body, your sense of self and your relationships. You may also start to wonder when to share your news. Give yourself time to allow the changes to settle into a new pattern.

Becoming a mum

The idea of becoming a mother takes some getting used to. Thankfully, it doesn't happen instantly; you have nine months to get used to the idea. During the pregnancy you'll probably begin to think about your own experiences as a child, and about people who have mothered you in your life (your own mum, certainly, but also people who have been motherly towards you). If these experiences were positive, you may decide to emulate those people and use them as role models; if they were negative, you may make a conscious decision to parent differently. Usually this is a gradual evolution as you begin the transition from the role of care-receiver to care-giver. Your new identity as a mother doesn't become fully cemented until well after the baby is born, so you've got plenty of time to figure it out.

> Time to go public, everyone: the pea is in the pod. I repeat, the pea is in the pod! #sprogged

If you find yourself worrying a lot, remind yourself that it's all part of the process. Like all rites of passage, you'll find that as you go through the pregnancy over the course of nine months, you'll become increasingly ready for your new role. Many women find it helpful to write their thoughts in a journal (read more on page 15). This is also a great time to take up meditation, which has been proven to help lower blood pressure and reduce stress levels. We'll discuss the actual how-to of meditation on pages 44–47.

Your partner

Sharing the news with a partner may be one of the most intimate moments of your life. Once you have, be aware that your partner will also start questioning his or her own capability as a future parent. Some partners need a while to warm up to the idea, while others are ready to be deeply involved from the start. However your partner takes the news, try to recognize that this is a great change for both of you, and you'll both need time to adjust to the idea of parenthood.

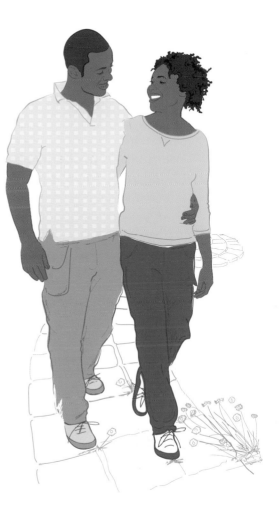

This is a great time to work on strengthening your relationship. During pregnancy, roles are more fluid, boundaries are open and identities start shifting, which gives you a unique opportunity to make lasting change in your life. If there are long-term issues that have plagued your relationship, now is a wonderful time to address them. Important life skills such as open communication and learning to fight 'fairly' will make the path to parenthood that much easier. It's also a good idea to try to recognize and discuss your own assumptions about parenting and domestic roles now, as these can turn out to be landmines after the birth.

Old family, new family

While most family members are thrilled at the idea of becoming grandparents, aunts and uncles, your impending motherhood will invariably force your family to see you in a new light. Sometimes it can be hard for parents to take a step back and give their daughter room to grow and develop into the kind of mother she wants to be. At other times you might be hoping for more help and support from your parents than they are able or willing to give. Navigating boundaries with a partner's family can also be tricky, and is often cited as a source of stress among new parents. Your new roles are rooted in the quality of your current relationships, and pregnancy is a wonderful time to work on improving communication with your family, old and new. Sitting down and talking with your parents and partner's family about your expectations can be one of the best ways to get your new family off on the right foot.

Sharing the news

Given how strange and tentative the first few weeks of pregnancy can sometimes feel, you might be wondering when it's a good time to tell others about it. In fact, there is no right time – it's entirely up to you. Some couples choose to tell their close friends and families immediately, to share the excitement and effectively activate their support network. Others, often those who have struggled to become pregnant, feel more comfortable waiting until they have passed certain milestones – such as the end of the first trimester, when the chance of miscarriage decreases.

Occasionally tensions can arise when sharing the news. If for some reason your secret is not greeted with jubilation, try to recognize that there may be other issues at play which have nothing to do with you – your best friend may be worried that she's going to lose you once you're a mother; another friend may have been trying to get pregnant without success. It's important to hold on to your own sense of happiness but also to accept that others may react differently. Try to give them the time and space they need to adjust to your news. Good friends almost always come around.

Your pregnancy journal

No one need ever see what you write, so this can be a safe and effective method for expressing and releasing your worries. It also doubles as a fabulous way to chronicle the many changes that occur during the pregnancy.

You might want to try a journal-writing technique known as 'sentence stemming' which can help you realize your innermost thoughts and feelings about a topic. At the top of the page, write one of the sentence stems listed below, and then quickly write 7–10 endings to the sentence. Write whatever comes to mind, and don't censor or judge what you're writing. Often the most important insights come after you've already written down several answers and are reaching for another. Be open to whatever comes up for you, and don't be surprised if these initial thoughts change – pregnancy is a time of huge transition.

• When I first learned about my pregnancy, I felt...
• A child in our life will... to my relationship with my life partner.
• At this time, having a child will...
• The gifts I want to give my child are...
• What I can do now to nurture and love my child is...

condensed idea
Pregnancy will raise emotional issues in you, your partner and those around you

4 A baby in the making

In the first trimester, your baby grows from two cells to a foetus approximately the size of an apricot. Not bad for 12 weeks of work! During this incredible time, your baby is developing all of her parts and organs, and setting the stage for her future growth and maturation.

One plus one is one

Prior to fertilization, your body goes through its monthly dance of preparation: your uterine lining thickens and ripens, a tiny ovum is prepared, and friendly cervical secretions grease the path for any intrepid sperm which might happen along, just as they do every month. Only this time, instead of getting your period, you conceive! Sperm meets egg; a microscopic, brand new bundle of cells journeys down your fallopian tube and snuggles into the thick and velvety lining of your uterus, and *voilà* – you're pregnant!

Amazingly, out of the millions of sperm available after ejaculation, only a single sperm is actually able to penetrate through the outer layers of the egg and cause fertilization. Once the sperm has entered the egg, the 23 chromosomes (small packages of DNA, or genetically coded material) from your partner join with the 23 chromosomes you have provided, and in that very instant, a brand new entity is made, with 46 chromosomes that will act to pass on all sorts of hereditary traits. This unique genetic blueprint is used by your body to create an entirely unique individual.

The gender of your future baby is also determined in this moment, based on whether the winning sperm contained a Y sex chromosome (boy) or an X sex chromosome (girl).

From zero to 12 weeks

In the first 24 hours after fertilization, the newly formed two-celled organism takes a well-deserved break. This pattern will occur again and again during the pregnancy (and in your baby after birth). Periods of intense growth and development are followed by periods of rest and integration. After its short nap, the fertilized egg goes through a remarkable growth spurt, dividing into 64 cells by day three and nearly 500 cells by day five. Implantation occurs around day eight, and the fertilized egg begins to secrete the pregnancy hormone hCG, which helps maintain the thick lining of the uterus and prevents uterine

Will my baby be okay?

You're not the first woman in history to stare in disbelief at the positive pregnancy test, then fearfully think back to the night of overindulgence you had two weeks ago at your friend's birthday party, which took place before you even realized you were pregnant!

Thankfully, Mother Nature has some developmental tricks up her sleeve to protect growing foetuses before mums become aware of their existence. For one thing, alcohol, drugs and other teratogens (substances that can cause birth defects or abnormalities) have their greatest effect during organ development, and this doesn't begin in a foetus until week five. Prior to that, teratogens may cause a miscarriage, but not a malformed baby. We'll discuss this topic in more detail on pages 24–27, but for now, try to breathe a sigh of relief: most women are healthy, and the vast majority of foetuses form without problems or anomalies.

shedding (a.k.a. your period). Around this time you might also notice some light spotting, which is normal and sometimes mistaken for a period. Even though you're officially pregnant, you won't miss your period for about another week (the fourth week of the pregnancy – remember, we're counting weeks from when your last period began, not from the moment of conception).

During the next few weeks, a lot happens all at once. The fertilized egg develops into two distinct parts: one part will go on to become the embryo, while the other begins to form the placenta, which will support and nourish your baby throughout the pregnancy. By the end of week four, the fertilized egg is now officially an embryo (and the size of a grain of rice), and it begins to develop into three layers. The innermost layer, called

> Week 9, and there are toes already – can you believe that? Tiny, minuscule toes. #1stTri

the endoderm, will form your baby's digestive tract, liver, pancreas and bladder; the middle layer, known as the mesoderm, will form your baby's skeleton, muscle layer, connective tissue, genitalia, spleen and heart; the outer layer, called the ectoderm, will eventually turn into your baby's skin, nails, hair, mammary glands, teeth and ears. That's a whole lot of baby crammed into three tiny layers!

A new heartbeat

By the sixth week of the pregnancy, a primitive heart begins to beat, and a small, rudimentary circulatory system begins to form, complete with blood vessels and blood cells. The backbone also begins its formation now, with the development of the neural tube (which eventually forms the brain and spinal cord) and five to eight vertebrae. Folic acid is essential to the process at this point, so even though your prenatal vitamins might be hard to choke down (courtesy of your morning sickness), they're valuable in helping to prevent neural tube defects.

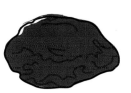

Week 4: your baby is the size of a grain of rice

Week 8: your baby reaches the size of a large cocktail olive

Week 10: growing fast, your baby becomes as large as a prune

Week 12: by the end of the first trimester, your baby is the size of an apricot

During the seventh to tenth week of pregnancy, your baby transforms from a small, tadpole-like creature to something that's recognizably human. The chest and abdomen form during the seventh week, and by week eight a small face and tiny rudimentary fingers and toes are visible. In the UK, the embryo is now officially recognized as a foetus (this occurs at week 10 in the USA). The formation of the baby's face, complete with eyelids, is finished by the ninth week. At ten weeks the circulatory system is really taking off: the heart has sped up from a rate of 80 beats per minute (bpm) to 120–160 bpm, major blood vessels are in place, and the external genitalia have even begun to differentiate.

By the end of the first trimester (12 weeks since your last period) the foetus is the size of an apricot, and all the body parts and major organs have formed. The muscles respond to brain signals, and the foetus is beginning to stretch and move on his own. He can even swallow and ball his hands into fists. The major organs will continue to mature in the months to come, but in 12 short weeks your baby has come a very long way indeed.

Condensed idea
By the end of week 12 your baby is fully formed

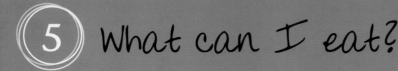

5 What can I eat?

If ever there was a time in your life when you really need to watch what you eat, this is it! Pregnancy is the perfect time to establish the healthy eating habits you will want to instil in your child, and everything you eat now is being used to form her bones and muscles.

Fresh and colourful

During pregnancy, three general rules for eating apply. First, fresh is always better than tinned or frozen. Second, try to 'eat the rainbow' (fruits and vegetables of every colour and hue, the more the better). Third, protein is your new best friend. Amazingly, to gain the right amount of weight, you need only 200–300 extra calories a day. This is equivalent to one extra serving of yogurt (containing 2 per cent milk fat), or one extra muesli bar, or two glasses of skimmed milk plus an apple and an egg. You need a whopping 60 g (2 oz) of protein a day, so fill up on eggs, lean meats, beans and legumes, tofu and soy products, nuts and nut-butters, and low-fat milk and milk products (Greek-style yogurt is a fantastic source of protein). Try to add a colourful salad to every meal, and have lots of fresh fruit with breakfast. You also need extra calcium (1200 mg daily) to form your baby's bones and teeth. You can get this from four glasses of milk, 45 g (1.5 oz) of hard cheese or 245 g (8 fl oz) plain yogurt.

Be a snacker

You'll probably find you have a much better time if you nibble and graze throughout the day than if you try to cram all of your calories into two or three large meals. In the first trimester this makes sense because you're often nauseous and not in the mood to eat much, and in the third trimester the baby is taking up all of the room your stomach would otherwise use to expand. Try to carry a few snacks with you wherever you go, to keep your blood-sugar levels steady and prevent spells of dizziness and lethargy. Examples of good snacks include apples with peanut butter, cheese and crackers, a yogurt and a piece of fruit, a muesli bar and a piece of fruit, a smoothie or some trail mix.

Supplements

If you're eating well, you're probably already gaining most of the nutrients you need to support a healthy pregnancy. Nevertheless, taking a good prenatal vitamin supplement during the pregnancy will ensure that you're getting enough of everything. Most over-the-counter prenatal vitamins have similar ingredients lists, which need to include at least 400 mcg of folic acid.

Foods to avoid

Surprisingly, the list is not as long as you might expect. Always practise proper food handling: wash all fruits and veggies before cooking; wash your hands thoroughly after handling raw meat; and make sure all meat is cooked thoroughly until there's no trace of pink or blood.

• Raw cheese or milk – the concern here is listeria, which can cause miscarriage, stillbirth and severe illness in newborns. Opt for cheese that says 'pasteurized' on its label. Cooked cheese (fondue, baked Brie or Camembert) is fine, because heating the cheese kills the bacteria. Some experts also recommend heating up cold cuts of meat in the microwave before eating as well.

• Sushi and pâté – for the same reasons as above.

• Raw or undercooked eggs – the risk here is salmonella poisoning.

• Fish high in mercury – especially tuna, mackerel, swordfish, shark and marlin. This is because mercury can harm the nervous system of a developing baby. Limit your intake of tuna to two steaks (or four small cans) a week and other oily fish (such as mackerel, sardines and trout) to two portions a week.

• Shellfish, unless thoroughly cooked and eaten instantly.

• More than 2 cups of coffee a day (more than 200 mg of caffeine a day). One brewed cup of coffee contains approximately 137 mg, tea 48 mg, soft drinks 37 mg, hot cocoa 8–12 mg.

• Liver – a very high source of vitamin A, and you're probably already getting plenty of this vitamin already.

If you're anaemic, your doctor or midwife may ask you to take additional iron. Be sure to take it at a different time from your prenatal vitamin, since the magnesium in the general vitamin tablet would prevent iron from being absorbed (but do drink down your iron tablet with a glass of orange juice, since vitamin C enhances absorption).

New research also suggests that supplementation with DHA (a type of omega-3 fatty acid) during pregnancy can help foetal brain development. Very few prenatal vitamins include DHA, so look for a separate supplement of 300–600 mg daily, preferably derived from algae, rather than fish oil (which may be contaminated by mercury and has been shown to thin the blood). Several European governments now advise pregnant women to take a vitamin D3 supplement, as a lack of sun in northern countries can lead to a deficiency of this vital bone-building vitamin.

> Hmmm, grapefruit with mustard… is actually really good. Who knew? #cravings

If you do decide to take supplements, remember that taking a prenatal vitamin is not a replacement for healthy eating, and bear in mind that it is possible to over-supplement. Vitamin A, for example, can cause foetal malformation in high amounts (more than 10,000 IUs daily). Read the label on your prenatal vitamin to make sure it does not contain vitamin A (sometimes present in the form of retinol). Excessive vitamin C during pregnancy can also be harmful to your baby, so avoid taking high doses (more than 80 mg a day) even if you're coming down with a cold.

Condensed idea
Although smelly blue cheeses, raw meat and wine are off the menu, luckily chocolate is still fine

6 Complete no-go's

You're not a fragile porcelain doll capable of breaking at any moment during pregnancy, but there are a few things you need to avoid and areas you need to be careful about. This chapter focuses on the most seriously harmful substances during pregnancy.

Caffeine, alcohol and tobacco

Most women know that tobacco and alcohol are off-limits even before they become pregnant, but they may not consider the effects of caffeine. This is the most common drug used by women worldwide as a quick 'pick-me-up', but while you're pregnant, it's best to limit caffeine intake to two cups of brewed coffee a day – at most. It is possible to be addicted to caffeine, so if you find you're having difficulty cutting back, or are experiencing withdrawal symptoms such as headaches, irritability and lethargy, speak to your doctor.

Many women enjoy a glass of wine, but drinking too much alcohol during pregnancy can lead to Foetal Alcohol Syndrome (which causes poor growth, mental retardation, behavioural issues and an abnormal facial appearance). The problem is, doctors don't know exactly how much alcohol is too much, so the general recommendation is not to drink any at all while you're pregnant or trying to conceive. Some medics believe that a glass of wine every now and then in the third trimester is fine, but talk this over with your own doctor and see what he or she suggests. As a general rule, alcohol and pregnancy do not mix!

The same goes for cigarettes. Here the advice is: while you're pregnant, don't smoke. Obviously smoking isn't good for you at any time, but while you're pregnant, your baby is essentially breathing through your bloodstream, so whatever you breathe in, he does too. in addition, when a woman smokes cigarettes (or breathes second-hand smoke), her blood contains significantly less oxygen, because some of it is replaced by chemicals such as carbon monoxide. In a pregnant woman, this can potentially result in

> I can live without the booze, but nine months without sushi? *gulp* #fishlover

poor growth of the baby, premature birth and developmental delays in the baby after birth, especially if smoke is inhaled during times of peak brain formation. Brains need oxygen, big time!

If you're a smoker, there's never been a better time to quit, and many women find that pregnancy is just the motivation they need to finally break their addiction. If you're having difficulty quitting, ask your doctor for a referral to a 'Quit Smoking' programme.

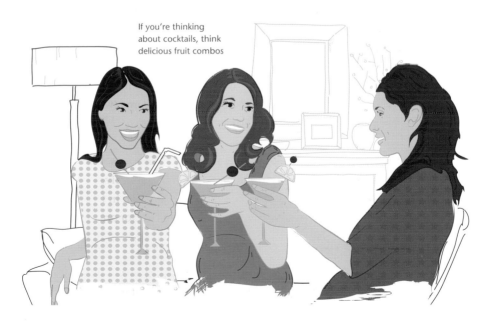

If you're thinking about cocktails, think delicious fruit combos

What about my cats?

Cats are the host animal for a parasite that causes toxoplasmosis, which can lead to miscarriage or severe foetal infection. Cats pick it up from eating infected mice or digging through the soil, and the parasite is released as spores in the cat's faeces. The risk of catching this is very rare, but limit your exposure by the following tips:

- Ask someone else to change the cat litter, or if you must do the deed yourself, use gloves and wash your hands with soap and water immediately afterwards.
- Scoop the litter regularly; it takes 2 days for cat faeces to become infectious – if you scoop frequently, you'll avoid the infectious stage altogether.
- Don't let your cat go outside, and avoid feeding your cat raw meat that may be contaminated.

Prescription drugs

Some prescription drugs are capable of causing birth defects, such as isotretinoin (Roaccutane), tetracycline, warfarin, streptomycin, gentamicin, chemotherapy agents and some cardiac medicines. Other medications, such as anticonvulsants, thyroid treatments, steroids and antidepressants, may have benefits that outweigh the risks. Make sure that all your healthcare providers are aware of every medication you're currently taking, and if you don't know whether it's safe during pregnancy, stop taking it until you find out for sure. If you have been taking an oral contraceptive, stop as soon as you find out that you are pregnant. As for over-the-counter medications, paracetamol (acetaminophen) is safe during pregnancy in low doses (the dose prescribed on the box), but all other pain medicines (including ibuprofen and aspirin) should be avoided.

Environmental and work hazards

Some industries, such as dry-cleaning, printing, manufacturing, and the aerospace and semiconductor industries, may expose you to harmful chemicals as part of your daily grind. Work exposure to chemicals, such as paint thinners, floor cleaners and glue, have the potential to cause foetal malformation and miscarriage. Ideally, avoid exposure to these chemicals altogether. If you must come into contact with them, use personal protective equipment at all times, ensure there is adequate ventilation, and limit exposure as much as possible. One other area to be aware of is potential harm from high lead levels, either from drinking water that runs through older (pre-1977) pipes, or as an occupational hazard (particularly plumbing, pipe fitting, auto repair, mining, glass manufacture, printing, refining or steel welding).

Street drugs

Opiates, cocaine, amphetamines and hallucinogens are all extremely dangerous during pregnancy and should be avoided at all costs. Opiates cause physical addiction in your baby, and cocaine is known to cause low birth weight, miscarriage, stroke, placental abruption (rupture), premature birth and even congenital malformations. Likewise, stimulants such as crystal meth (methamphetamine) lead to low birth weight, prematurity, cleft palate, developmental delays and miscarriage. Hallucinogens such as LSD can cause abnormalities in a baby's development. Like tobacco, marijuana may lead to decreased blood oxygenation and low birth weight, and has been shown to adversely affect foetal brain development. Marijuana also increases the harmful effects of alcohol, and may increase the likelihood of foetal alcohol syndrome.

Condensed idea
Don't take any form of drug without checking first with your doctor

7 Looking after yourself

Taking care of yourself is also the best way to take care of your baby, and you'll probably find that it feels particularly satisfying during pregnancy. Small treats sprinkled throughout your day can help make you feel happier, more secure and surprisingly content.

Breast and belly care

The kindest gift you can give to your tender and growing breasts is a comfy and supportive bra. Your breasts will probably increase by at least one cup size during the pregnancy, and then another cup size again once you're nursing. Towards the end of the pregnancy, you may choose to buy a nursing bra rather than another larger-sized regular bra. Nursing bras are usually soft-structured rather than underwired, with flaps that fold down to allow easy access to your nipples. If you're unsure about the size, generally buy one cup size up from what you're currently wearing towards the end of your pregnancy.

Unfortunately, there's no product you can buy that will prevent stretch marks (although there are many that claim otherwise!). Stretch marks are caused by genetics – either you'll get them or you won't. You'll probably also notice a line of darker pigmentation running down the centre of your belly as the pregnancy progresses. This is called the linea nigra, and it's a normal skin change that fades away completely several months after the birth.

Amazingly, research has shown that babies are soothed when the mother rubs her belly (in fact pregnant women often unconsciously do this from about 23 weeks on), so using a natural moisturizer – such as cocoa butter

– every evening as part of your bedtime routine can be a relaxing ritual for both of you, while helping to keep your skin soft and supple too.

As your belly grows larger, you may also find that an abdominal support or pregnancy girdle can help relieve lower back and ligament pain, although it won't actually prevent loss of muscle tone (thankfully,

Travelling with your bump

Travelling is safe during pregnancy, but always take a copy of your antenatal records with you – just in case – and bear the following points in mind:

- The second trimester is the best time to plan major trips – you're out of the danger zone for miscarriage but still far from the actual due date.
- Check with your airline before you leave; they may require a medical authorization or may limit flying past a certain number of weeks.
- Request an aisle seat when flying so you'll have extra leg room to stretch out.
- Get up and walk around the cabin every hour or so. Air travel increases your risk of deep vein thrombosis (DVT), as does pregnancy, but leg movement decreases the risk.
- Avoid visiting malarial regions and places with ongoing outbreaks of life-threatening infections borne by food or insects.
- Check beforehand whether blood for transfusions is screened for HIV and Hepatitis B at your destination country.

your normal abdominal tone is pretty much back to where you started by 10 weeks after the birth, and can be strengthened even more with abdominal exercises at that point).

Dental care

Good dental hygiene is crucial, especially as your gums bleed more easily and are more sensitive during pregnancy, which increases the risk of gingivitis and periodontal infections, and can even lead to premature birth. Brushing twice a day and having at least one dental check-up and polish during the pregnancy can help prevent this (dental care is free during pregnancy

> Just left the bathroom looking like a defeated boxer. Tired, nauseous and now bleeding gums? #notallfun

with the NHS), but try to have major dental work done either before or after the pregnancy. Tell your dentist that you're pregnant so that he or she can adjust treatment accordingly. In general, local anaesthetics like lidocaine are safe during pregnancy, but stronger forms of anaesthesia like nitrous oxide ('laughing gas') or general anaesthesia should be avoided. Dental X-rays are okay if necessary, but it's better to avoid them in the first trimester if possible. Your dentist can cover your belly with a lead apron to help protect the foetus from the second trimester on.

Bathing

Raising your core body temperature during pregnancy has been associated with birth defects (especially in the first trimester), so sadly saunas and hot tubs are off limits during pregnancy. Showering is fine, of course, and a nice soak in water cooler than 37.7°C (100°F) is a fantastic daily or weekly treat. When washing, there's no need to use any special soaps when cleaning the vulva and vagina. Resist any urge to douche, too – the vagina is self-cleaning, and douching destroys the normal bacterial flora which keeps the vagina healthy.

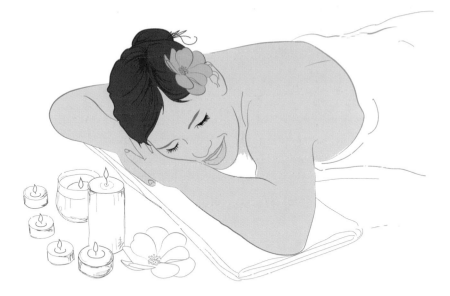

Treat yourself

Stress relief is more important during pregnancy than at any other time in your life, so build plenty of relaxation and treats into your week. Long, luxurious bath? Check. Manicure or pedicure? Absolutely (although make sure the salon is well-ventilated). Book yourself one or two (or several) prenatal massages, but avoid aromatherapy massages: some essential oils can cause problems, so it's safest to steer clear completely. Sleepy? Go ahead and take that extra nap. Feel like a nibble? Treat yourself to some dark chocolate (full of antioxidants, and possibly reduces your risk of pre-eclampsia later in the pregnancy). Whatever you do to unwind and relax, make sure you do it often.

Condensed idea
Pregnancy is a great time to take extra-special care of yourself

8 Keep it moving

Get on up! Research shows that exercise in pregnancy helps with those pesky symptoms (swollen ankles, backache, constipation), improves your posture and muscle tone, and even helps build endurance – something you'll need for your upcoming marathon event!

The new thinking

Exercise in pregnancy used to be actively discouraged, but today it's quite the opposite situation. Research shows that all of the normal benefits of exercise still apply during pregnancy, only more so. It helps combat fatigue and low energy, especially during the first and

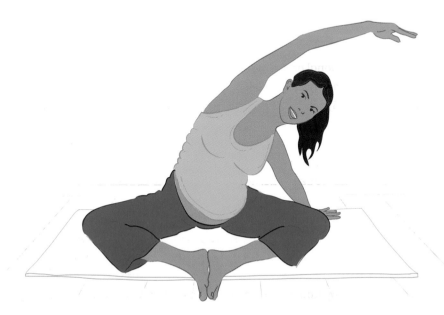

third trimesters when lethargy is at its worst. The endorphins released during exercise will also help lift your mood and reduce stress, depression and anxiety.

Stretching and moving helps relieve many of the aches and pains of pregnancy, such as lower back pain, round ligament pain and sciatica, and can even help with constipation (moving your body helps move your bowels). Exercise helps promote deeper and more restful sleep, prevents excessive weight gain, and can even help fend off gestational diabetes.

Studies also show again and again that a fit mother makes a fit baby. When you exercise, your heart rate increases and your blood pressure temporarily rises – and your baby's does as well, which suggests that your baby receives all of the same cardiovascular benefits from exercise as you do. Babies born to women who exercise can recover from stress more quickly and tend to be born at healthier birth weights (not too big or too small). Fit mothers are likely to have a shorter labour and a faster postnatal recovery, and they're less likely to need a caesarian section.

Get the all-clear first

This might seem like an unnecessary step, especially when all of the most professional organizations (such as the Royal College of Obstetricians and Gynaecologists in the UK and the American College of Obstetrics and Gynecology in the USA) are advising daily work-outs, but before you begin any exercise programme, check in with your midwife or healthcare provider first. Make sure they're aware of your normal exercise routine and current fitness level so you're both on the same page; your idea of 'moderate' might be very different from theirs.

Exercise is still discouraged if you're experiencing any rare pregnancy complications, such as premature labour, cervical incompetence, foetal growth restriction or pregnancy-induced high blood pressure. If you are having a healthy pregnancy, though, there's probably no reason you can't exercise – up until the day you go into labour, if you like!

How much is enough?

Moderation is the name of the game. Pregnancy is not the time to start any rigorous new programmes or endurance training, but if you already have a regular exercise routine, your doctor will probably encourage you to stick to that. Never work out to the point of exhaustion – stop when you become fatigued, or take it down a notch. Try the talk test: if you're unable to talk while you're exercising, you're exerting yourself too much. If you exercise too strenuously or for too long, your temperature will rise, and

The do's and don'ts of exercising

- Do keep yourself well hydrated – drink before, during and after every workout.
- Do wear loose, comfortable and breathable clothing.
- Do eat a small and nourishing snack about an hour before your work-out to keep your energy levels up.
- Do slow down and take your time, especially as your ligaments soften in the third trimester and your belly gets bigger.
- Do stop immediately if you have bleeding, cramping, loss of fluid, chest tightness, dizziness or pain.
- Don't exercise outside on hot and humid days; it's much easier to overheat when you're pregnant.
- Don't lie flat on your back for extended periods of time in the second and third trimester – the weight of your belly can compress the main vein next to your spine and limit blood-flow to the placenta.
- Don't overdo it. Make sure you can always breathe and speak easily.

your baby's temperature – which is already higher than your own – will rise too, which may cause a problem for the baby. So don't overdo it, and take it down another notch if you're in a hot or humid place. In addition, always make sure that any fitness instructor you use knows how many weeks pregnant

> So lovely swimming now that the bump is getting bigger. #fitmum

you are. In general, 30 minutes (or slightly more) of moderate exercise is recommended on most days, but this can be broken up into 10-minute chunks. Even simple things like gardening or choosing to take the stairs at work instead of the lift can be a decent work-out. Just remember to keep yourself well hydrated while you're exercising, wear a supportive bra and appropriate shoes, and listen to your body: if you can't catch your breath, feel faint or dizzy, or are experiencing any pain, stop!

Keep it simple

It probably goes without saying, but pregnancy is not the time to play contact sports like rugby or football, or to do anything with the potential for falling, such as climbing, horse riding or skiing. Even activities which you might be used to doing regularly might become more difficult during pregnancy as your centre of gravity shifts with your burgeoning bump, so check in with your body frequently. Low-impact sports are your best bet, and thankfully there are lots of them: swimming, walking or biking (especially on a stationary bike – less chance of falling). Sign up for a class which looks interesting to you, such as prenatal yoga or pilates, and you might even make a few new friends along the way.

Condensed idea
Keeping fit and healthy will make childbirth easier for you and your baby

9 A working mum

More women are now employed outside the home than ever before, and the workplace is becoming more family-friendly than ever. Many women choose to work right up until the moment they go into labour, which is fine if you're taking good care of yourself at work.

Pregnancy on the job

Work and pregnancy can sometimes be a difficult mix, especially as you cope with physical symptoms, emotional roller-coasters, and having to get to your frequent medical appointments. Do yourself a favour and try to arrive at work every morning with a full tummy, lots of snacks to nibble on throughout the day, plenty of hydrating drinks, and comfortable work clothing and shoes (especially if you have to stand for long stretches). Most jobs are safe to continue to do while pregnant, especially if your job is in an office or at a desk. If you are desk-bound, it's a good idea to change position fairly regularly and stretch your legs, which will help avoid those pregnancy aches and pains and prevent deep vein thrombosis (or DVT – blood clots in the lower leg). Intense physical exertion, such as standing in one place for hours at a time, heavy lifting and long work hours, has been associated with a slightly higher risk of premature delivery, so if you have a job like that, take lots of breaks and make sure you keep hydrated.

Do your research

What you're entitled to in terms of maternity leave varies considerably from country to country, so it's important to find out exactly what's available, and what you may have to do to secure it. In the UK, a woman

Work–life balance

The work–life balance gets even harder to juggle with a baby as opposed to a bump, so your pregnancy is a good opportunity to practise the balancing act. Here are a few tips to make it work:

- If nausea is an issue, bring lots of crackers and snacks with you, and nibble throughout the day.
- If your co-workers' lunch smells are turning your stomach, eat on your own, or go outside for lunch.
- Pack a comfort bag with everything you might need in case you vomit: a clean top, a washcloth, a toothbrush, mints or gum.
- Schedule regular standing and stretching breaks into your day – ideally every hour, perhaps at the same time as a toilet break.
- Prop your feet up under your desk – even a slight elevation helps relieve swelling and fatigue.
- Keep some extra sweaters and comfy shoes at work, as your body temperature can be unpredictable (hot feet swell!).

is entitled to 52 weeks of maternity leave, regardless of how long she has been with her employer, how many hours she works a week or how much she is paid, as long as she is classed as an 'employee' (check www.gov.uk if in doubt) and informs her employer of the pregnancy at least 15 weeks before the baby is due. She is entitled to start maternity leave any time up to 11 weeks before the baby's due date, and will receive around 90 per cent of her salary for six weeks, then a lower, government-set amount for a further 33 weeks. In many countries, such as the UK, women are guaranteed to have a job to come back to if they give their employer full notice, but be sure to check the statutory conditions set out by your own firm and government. Talk with your human resources department, read your employee handbook and discreetly ask other colleagues who've had babies about how the process works. The better informed you are, the easier your conversation with your boss will be.

Telling your boss

Just like breaking the news to your family and friends, sharing your secret with your boss is a very personal decision which depends greatly on your relationship with your boss, how family-friendly your company is, and how crucial your job is to the business as a whole. Most women tend to wait until the end of the first trimester, when the risk of miscarriage decreases, but if you're starting to show sooner than that or find yourself spending a lot of quality time in the toilets, you might think about sharing the news earlier. If your job is dangerous, incredibly stressful or demanding (24-hour shifts? night-call? on your feet 12 hours a day?) or exposes you to harmful chemicals, it's probably best to tell your employer right away, so you can minimize the potential danger.

If you have a very close and open relationship with your boss, you might decide to share your secret sooner as well, so you can take advantage of any benefits your company might have to offer pregnant women (such as flexible hours, working from home, or leaving early in the afternoons to get to medical appointments). On the other hand, if your company isn't very family-friendly, or you're fairly certain your boss won't take the news well, you might want to wait until 16–20 weeks to reveal the news (assuming you can hide it for that long). That way your boss will see that you're able to continue to meet the demands of your job during your pregnancy. Pick

Turned in the expense reports, nailed my presentation, peed 6 times, ate 7 snacks and no one even knows I'm pregnant! #workgoddess

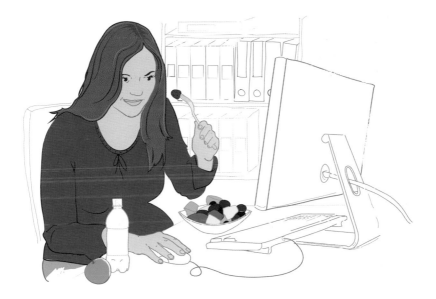

a time when both of you are not too overloaded with work or distracted, then present your boss with a plan on how you'll continue to handle your responsibilities while pregnant, together with ideas for how your work can be delegated to others while you're away.

The bigger picture

Many women use pregnancy as an opportunity to re-evaluate their career and life priorities; some stop work for a while or even change career. You'll need to think about how long you can take off work, whether your family can get by on one salary for a while or not, and any other emotional or logistical factors that might affect your decision – such as the demands of your job, child-care considerations, your commute, and when you think you'll be ready (or able) to leave your child to return to work again.

condensed idea
Know and claim all your pregnancy working rights!

10 Is this normal?

In the midst of all of the strange changes that are happening to your body while you're pregnant, it's sometimes hard to tell what's normal and what's not. Rest assured, if it's something that has just come up in the last few weeks, the pregnancy is probably to blame.

A lot going on down there

Given that it's the only part of your reproductive tract which you can actually see, it's not surprising that some of the biggest changes you'll notice appear between your legs. For one thing, you might see a lot more vaginal discharge than usual. These secretions come from the increased glandular activity of the cervix. It's called leukorrhoea (*leukos* is the Greek word for 'white', while *rhoia* means 'flow'), and so long as it's white, milky or creamy, with no strong odour or itchiness, it's a perfectly healthy thing. Of course, healthy doesn't necessarily mean mess-free, and many women decide to wear panty-liners during their pregnancy to protect their underwear. Just remember that douching is never a good idea (now or at any point) – it disrupts your normal, healthy bacterial balance, promotes infection, and can potentially cause an air embolism during pregnancy.

> Feels like I'm sitting in a lake, day and night – please tell me this is normal?!? #preggershelp

On the flip side, of course, if you have discharge which is itchy, yellow or green, frothy or curdy, or which has a bad smell, you've probably picked up a vaginal infection of some kind. These infections can occur

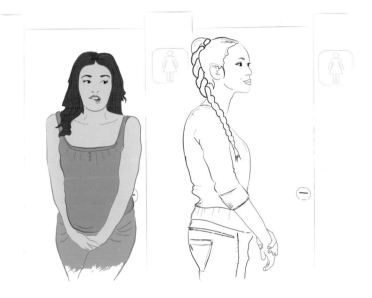

more frequently during pregnancy thanks to hormonal disruption of the delicate and finely tuned pH balance of the vagina. Luckily, they are easy to treat with medication, so ask your midwife or doctor to carry out checks.

Varicose veins can also occur in your vulva or vagina during pregnancy, just as they can in your legs. These usually present as soft blue cords running beneath the skin of the labia or vulva, sometimes knotted or lumpy looking. While often harmless, they can become tender or inflamed, especially if you're on your feet for long periods. The good news is that they generally go away after the pregnancy, but there's not much you can do in the meantime. Sometimes wearing a pair of pregnancy support tights can help.

Bladder matters

You're probably already well aware of the frequent peeing that happens during pregnancy, but you might be relieved to know that this is normal. In the first trimester it happens because the growing uterus is still housed in your pelvis, which means it's constantly putting pressure on your

Pregnancy and chronic illness

As more and more women are now delaying childbearing until later in life, the number of women entering pregnancy with chronic illness is also increasing.

Fortunately, many chronic diseases, such as high blood pressure, thyroid disorders, diabetes, heart disease, lupus and asthma can be managed concurrently in such a way that they don't negatively impact the pregnancy, and many women can have a totally normal and healthy pregnancy and birth. The key is making sure that the chronic illness is well controlled during the pregnancy. This sometimes means continuing on certain drug regimens because the risk of not being on the drug is much worse than the risk of using the drug during pregnancy (such as with epilepsy).

If you have a chronic illness, make sure you notify your midwife or doctor of your history as soon as you know you are pregnant (ideally, doctors should be informed while you're trying to get pregnant). Planning in advance is important to ensure a good outcome and to prevent any problems with medication.

poor bladder. It doesn't help that the pregnancy hormone hCG is also a diuretic – and your levels of this are highest in the first trimester as well. In the third trimester, the culprit is two-fold: increased blood volume leads to increased urination, and the baby's head starts to ride low in the pelvis around 34 weeks, applying pressure again. You also might notice more frequent urination at night as water from your swollen legs returns to your core, and your kidneys work overtime to get it processed.

However, any pain or burning with urination, in addition to frequency or an intense need to urinate *right now!* may be a sign of a urinary tract infection, or UTI. Unfortunately, these happen more frequently during pregnancy thanks to – you guessed it! – the hormonal changes taking place, which dilate and enlarge the kidneys and ureters. Treatment involves a course of antibiotics, which is usually sufficient to get rid of it. UTIs also cause

> Good to learn that peeing all the time in pregnancy is normal – I was getting concerned! #legscrossed

kidney infections much more easily when you're pregnant, and these can be quite serious, so if you notice any intense back pain, fever, chills or aching, call your midwife or doctor. It may be serious enough to require a hospital admission and IV antibiotics, so don't ignore the symptoms.

And all the rest

Sexually transmitted infections (STIs) are never normal, but annoyingly, many of them are completely asymptomatic. In the UK, you will automatically be screened for HIV/AIDS and syphilis, but if you suspect any other form of sexually transmitted infection, you will need to visit a genito-urinary medicine clinic for full screening. Herpes is one virus that doctors can't cure, but they can at least cut down on its duration and frequency. If you have genital herpes, as long as you don't have an active outbreak at the time of delivery, you can still plan on a vaginal birth. The most important things to focus on with STIs is making sure your partner is treated as well, and making sure the infection doesn't come back.

Condensed idea
Many pregnancy symptoms are perfectly normal, even if they feel a bit unusual

(11) Happy and relaxed

Chronic stress has been proven to increase the risk of miscarriage and cause premature labour, so it's important during pregnancy to find ways to relax and unwind after anxious days or events. Try introducing relaxing and replenishing practices into your day.

The mother-baby connection

While all of this growth and development is miraculously going on inside you without any conscious thought on your part, recent research suggests that in fact there is a huge connection between mother and baby, and that your emotional state during the pregnancy forms the backbone of your baby's temperament. According to US doctor and author Dr Frederick Wirth, whatever you feel, the baby also feels, thanks to the passage of neuropeptides across the placental barrier. These neuropeptides carry emotional messages, such as stress, fear or contentment, and your baby responds to these neuropeptides in the same way as you do.

The important take-away message here is not to try to prevent stress at all costs (an impossible feat) or to worry unduly if you do become stressed (worrying about avoiding it will just make you more stressed), but to recognize that every time you feel stressed, the next step is to take a moment to consciously relax. This will send a message of calm and security to your developing baby. Imagine, for instance, that you're driving down the road, then another car suddenly pulls out in front of you. The surge in adrenaline and the heart-pounding fear you feel as you slam on the brakes are also experienced by your baby. Afterwards, knowing that you have avoided a crash, you realize (rationally) that

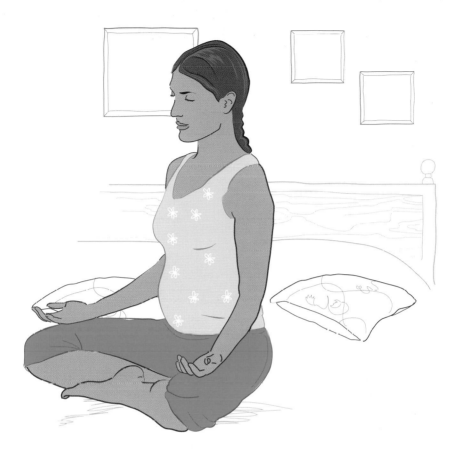

you're okay, but your baby still has no idea that he can relax. All he knows is your fear and panic, without understanding the reason behind it. That's why it's so important to take a few deep breaths to relax your body and tell your baby: 'Wow! That was scary, but we're all right now.'

Your baby is aware of everything you're saying to him. He might not understand the words themselves, but he feels the intention behind them. Studies have shown again and again that he will recognize your voice immediately when he's born, and that it will relax and comfort him. So even though it might feel silly at this point, talk to your baby throughout your day. Always acknowledge him as your companion as you go about your business. Sing your baby a song, or soothe her after you've had a stressful moment. She will feel your love, so be sure to give her plenty of loving attention while she's literally bathing in your emotional state.

Stress antidotes

Stress releases adrenaline, while peace and contentment release oxytocin, the hormone of love, so it's vital that you find ways to unwind during your pregnancy. Exercise is a fantastic way to do this (see more on pages 32–35), because it releases a cocktail of feelgood endorphins that are known to elevate mood and improve a sense of wellbeing. Yoga is also a proven method of stress relief (with exercise thrown in as a bonus), and is a wonderful practice for pregnant women. Kissing, hugging and snuggling all release oxytocin, as does having sex with a loving partner.

> Just nodded off while meditating – bliss before and after! #calmernow

'Grounding' is another technique you can do to quickly calm yourself (and your baby) after a stressful moment. To practise this, all you have to do is stop for a moment and feel the point where your body connects to the ground beneath you (your feet on the floor, or your bottom in your chair). Then take a deep breath and focus on that grounding point. Meditation is another great way to clear your mind and relax, with proven health benefits thrown in to boot (see box, opposite). If that's too esoteric for you, though, try walking barefoot in a park every now and then – it might sound silly, but it will probably relax you! This practice is known as 'earthing', and some practitioners believe it's a great way to reconnect ourselves to the healing energies of the earth, helping to stabilize our electrical systems and maintain our health. If it feels good, and it's safe for baby, do it. And make sure you build plenty of pampering into your week – see pages 28–31 for ideas on little treats. Even very small things, like a square of chocolate, can release oxytocin.

Meditation for beginners

Like anything, the key to meditation is practice. You'll probably not get it on your first (or 10th) try, but keep at it and you'll be amazed at how 10–15 minutes a day can really make a difference.

- Find a comfortable position. If you're a beginner, you might have better luck sitting, as you'll probably drop off to sleep if you're lying down.
- Close your eyes and picture a gentle rippling stream or a deep, blue underwater scene.
- Let your thoughts flow through your mind unhindered. It's impossible to stop thinking, but just observe your thoughts as they occur, rather than respond to them.
- Picture your thoughts floating down the rippling stream like leaves on water, or like bubbles rising in your underwater scene. Let each thought present itself, then acknowledge it and allow your mind to float off again without dwelling on it.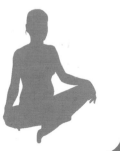
- If you find yourself getting stuck, simply move back to your stream or watery depths, and let go of all your thoughts.
- Practice, practice, practice! Start off with five minutes a day, then move to 10 or 15.

condensed idea
Consciously practising relaxation techniques will keep you happy and your pregnancy healthier

12 Testing, testing

Unfortunately, prenatal care involves a lot of testing, which can be very difficult if you're scared of needles. But understanding the reasoning behind the tests can make you feel less like a human pin-cushion and more like an active participant in your antenatal care.

Antenatal care

The purpose of antenatal care is to produce better pregnancy outcomes – this means fewer maternal and newborn health problems. However, antenatal care isn't just about your health: it's also designed to prepare you mentally for birth; support you throughout your pregnancy, birth and postnatal period; and help you develop parenting skills and support structures. That's a lot of care crammed into nine short months!

The actual tests performed will vary based on your current health, age, location, and whether any complications occur during the pregnancy. The next few pages explain the routine tests that are most often

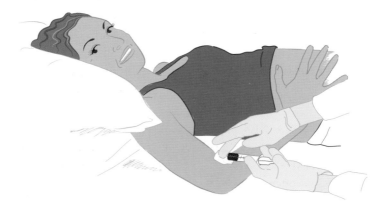

performed, but don't be concerned if your doctor includes additional tests or doesn't perform all of those listed here. Good antenatal care is tailored to your individual needs.

First trimester tests

At the initial visit, your doctor will take your health history, perform a thorough physical examination and take blood and urine samples. Your blood will provide the medical team with important information. First, it is used to establish your blood type and Rh factor, to check for potential incompatibility between your blood and the baby's blood (this is very important if you're Rh Negative – for more on this see page 76). Second, your blood count will show if you are suffering from anaemia and whether you have a normal platelet count (this is important for adequate blood clotting after the birth). Third, it can also be used to check for infection; pregnant women are routinely tested for Hepatitis B, syphilis and HIV, to allow treatment if necessary. Several routine genetic carrier screening tests are also performed, including sickle cell disease and thalassaemia (in the USA they test for cystic fibrosis too), and more specialized screens may be performed in cases of possible higher risk (read more on genetic testing on pages 68–71). Your blood test will also show if you're immune to rubella, or German measles; if not, the vaccine can be given after the birth. In some countries your lead level may also be checked, as high levels can cause birth defects. Finally, your urine will probably be checked for signs of infection, particularly urinary tract infections.

> Just heard her tiny heart for the first time – it was love at first beat.
> #wildaboutthebabe

An early ultrasound scan may be done to help date the pregnancy (especially if you're unsure of the date of your last period), confirm that the foetus is in the uterus (in an ectopic pregnancy the foetus develops outside the uterus, often in a fallopian tube) and to determine whether

Anatomy of an antenatal visit

Your average antenatal visit will probably include the following elements:

- Your weight and blood pressure will be checked, and a urine sample will be dipped.
- Your healthcare professional will ask if you have any new complaints or symptoms.
- Your healthcare professional will make sure you're feeling the baby move regularly (if applicable), and will ask about vaginal bleeding, cramping or loss of fluid.
- The size of your baby will be measured and you'll listen to your baby's heart beat.
- Your healthcare professional will update you with the results of any tests or scans you may have had since the last visit.
- You'll have an opportunity to discuss any of your concerns – remember, nothing is off limits!
- Any blood needed for tests will be drawn or scheduled to be drawn, and your next follow-up visit will be arranged. Usually the visits are every month up until 28–32 weeks, then every two weeks after that up until 36 weeks, then weekly from 36 weeks on.

you're carrying twins or not. If you opt for further genetic tests, such as CVS (chorionic villus sampling), these are usually done 10–13 weeks into the pregnancy (read more on page 70). You may feel slightly anxious as you wait for this first raft of test results to come back, but the majority of women will receive reassuring results and after they're back you'll probably be relieved to know you were thoroughly checked.

Second trimester tests

Testing eases off as you come into the second trimester. If you declined genetic testing in the first trimester, however, you can opt to do it in the second. In the UK blood tests may be drawn at any time from 10–20 weeks to check for Down's syndrome, Trisomy 18 and neural tube defects (read more on pages 68–69). This is also the trimester in which you will have a detailed ultrasound scan (or 'foetal anomaly screening'), at around 18–21 weeks to check foetal development, organ growth, placental location and amniotic fluid volume (it can also tell you the gender of your baby, if you want to know!). At around week 28 your haemoglobin levels may be checked again, as this is the point in the pregnancy when some women start to become anaemic. You will also be checked for gestational diabetes, which sometimes develops in pregnancy.

Third trimester tests

By the third trimester, you're usually on cruise control, with little testing or interference by medical staff. Any earlier issues will probably have been dealt with and any tests now are usually follow-up tests to those done earlier. Based on how your pregnancy is progressing, you may continue to have follow-up ultrasounds or blood tests. As you near the delivery date your doctor may repeat tests for STIs and take swabs to test for Group B Streptococcus (GBS). In the UK, screening for GBS is offered only if a doctor feels it is indicated. GBS is a normal bacteria which is found in around 30 per cent of all women, and it's rare for babies to become infected with it, but if they do it can become very serious. If GBS is present at the time of birth, you'll be given intravenous antibiotics. It's worth remembering that all these tests are aimed at protecting you and your baby.

Condensed idea
Antenatal care helps ensure the best possible outcome for you and your baby

13 Surprise!

It's not impossible that as you settle in for your first ultrasound scan, you'll hear, 'Oh look, twins!' Pregnancy, like life, is known for throwing curve balls. The good news is that it's all just a practice run for parenting, which you will soon discover is full of surprises.

Am I likely to have twins?

There are two types of twins. Identical twins occur when a fertilized egg divides very early in its development, whereas fraternal twins occur when two eggs are released by the mother and both are fertilized at the same time. Identical twins contain all of the same genetic material, whereas fraternal twins are basically siblings born at the same time.

With the increase in IVF and other fertility treatments, the prevalence of twins, triplets or more is rising. If you became pregnant through a fertility treatment, you are probably well aware of how many babies you're carrying. In the general population, a woman's chance of spontaneously conceiving twins is still approximately 1 in 90 (in some populations as high as 1 in 42), and it's even higher if there are twins running in your family – especially on your mother's side – or if you're in your late 30s or older.

Antenatal care for multiples

When you first find out you're carrying multiple babies, your first reaction might be shock, followed by anxiety about their wellbeing or how you're going to manage to parent more than one baby at the same time. While twins and other multiples have the potential for twice as much fun, they do face greater risks and challenges during pregnancy. The chance of prematurity is much higher than it is with singleton pregnancies. There is also a slightly higher chance of problems developing with the placenta during twin gestation; sometimes one twin receives a greater share of blood than the other (known as twin-to-twin transfusion syndrome). Having twins also increases the risk of problems for the mother, who stands a greater chance of developing pre-eclampsia, gestational diabetes and anaemia. For all of these reasons, twins are generally treated as a high-risk pregnancy – meaning that you'll receive extra care.

The good news

While all of this can sound alarming, the survival rate for twins is higher now than at any other point in history, and doctors and midwives are much better at taking care of twin pregnancies. Early ultrasound scans

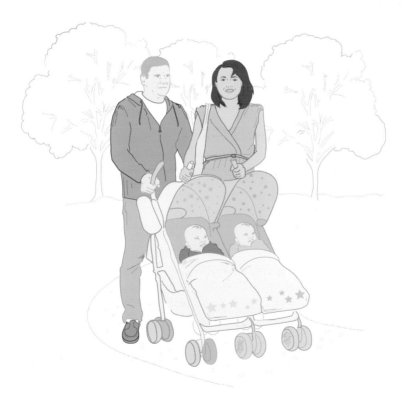

Economies of scale

There are at least 10 reasons why having twins is brilliant:

- If you were thinking you wanted more than one child eventually, you've got it taken care of – in one fell swoop!
- Your babies will always have a built-in playdate: each other.
- Almost everything is cheaper in bulk, especially nappies and wipes.
- Once they're potty trained, you never have to deal with nappies again (unless you want to).
- You only have to get through one pregnancy for two babies (and who wants morning sickness more than once?).
- The best-friend benefit: you will be amazed by how well your babies will comfort and help each other.
- You never have to juggle a toddler and a baby at the same time – they're always the same age.
- You'll have a great team of little helpers: four hands to put to work instead of just two.
- A double pushchair holds a lot more shopping than a single one.
- You'll become the most organized person you know – because you have to be!

mean that multiples are often detected in the first trimester, giving you plenty of time to optimize your health and prepare for the birth. You'll also probably have an entire team helping you out. While your obstetrician or midwife are likely to remain your primary care providers, they will probably be in consultation with a perinatologist (a specialist in high-risk pregnancy) and possibly a neonatologist (a specialist in newborn babies) or paediatrician (a specialist in child heath) as well, once the delivery draws closer. This team is there to ensure that your twosome (or threesome, or foursome) will be very closely monitored, and any complications can be dealt with promptly.

While many of the discomforts of pregnancy might be twice as uncomfortable (lower back pain, anyone? And don't even mention those poor swollen ankles!), there's a good chance that you'll have an uncomplicated delivery. Sometimes a caesarean is required, but if both babies have their heads down by the end of the pregnancy, you may be able to have a totally natural vaginal delivery (well, two of them, technically).

> TWO heart beats on the ultrasound today! Um…HELP?! #shockandawe

Going with the flow

There are plenty of other complications of pregnancy which can throw you for a loop. Being diagnosed with gestational diabetes, for instance, or discovering that you'll need months of bed-rest or a caesarean for some reason. Sometimes it helps to keep your eye on the big picture – healthy mum, healthy baby(ies) – rather than the specific details. Remembering that there are plenty of factors beyond your control can also help give you a wider perspective. It can be hard to let go of something that may have been a part of your birth plan, but once you can lay it to rest, you'll find plenty of positives to enjoy. This is your journey, after all, and these surprises are just bumps in the road.

Condensed idea
Twins or more mean you'll have lots of extra attention, but not necessarily any more complications

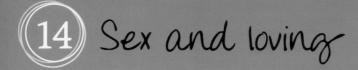

(14) Sex and loving

You might be pleased to learn that sex while pregnant is normal and healthy, and definitely allowed. Or you might find yourself feeling anything but sexy – and this is normal, too. Whatever your feelings are, be sure to keep up the communication with your partner.

A few adjustments

Pregnancy hormones don't affect everyone in the same way – some women find that they have absolutely no interest in sex during their entire pregnancy, while others are ravenous from day one, and both of these reactions are entirely normal (as is everything in between).

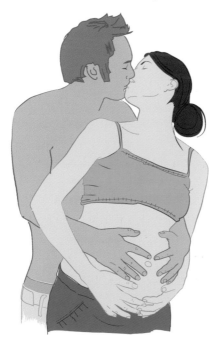

So relax – there are no hard and fast rules for libido in pregnancy. Many women find it difficult to feel sexy in their new, changing bodies, especially in the later trimesters as they start to gain more weight. Sometimes it helps to remind yourself that this is temporary, or to buy a new top or dress that flatters your curves and makes you feel sexy, bump and all.

You might also find yourself worrying about whether or not sex while pregnant can hurt the baby. In fact, the baby is actually very well protected behind

A word of caution

Before embarking on a night of passion, it's worth checking that you're physically able to do so! While rare, there are a few instances in pregnancy when sex definitely needs to be avoided, such as:

- If you have a low-lying placenta, or placenta previa (where the placenta has implanted over the cervix).
- If you break your bag of waters.
- If you've been having premature labour.
- If you're experiencing any heavy vaginal bleeding.
- If you've been having any problems with cervical incompetency, or have received a cervical stitch.
- If you or your partner have an untreated sexually transmitted infection. (Using condoms can help protect you from this, but they aren't 100 per cent reliable, so it's better to wait until you have both been treated.)
- If you have been diagnosed with a threatened miscarriage, or are experiencing any signs of a miscarriage, such as bleeding or cramping (see page 62 for more information).

your cervix by layers of muscle and fat, and cushioned in a balloon of amniotic fluid, so lovemaking (even the very vigorous kind) won't cause any actual harm. Research has also shown that in a healthy, low-risk pregnancy, sex doesn't cause or increase the risk of miscarriage or premature labour (although if you're already having problems with premature labour, sex may potentially make it worse, so avoid it if that's the case).

Your partner might also experience some changes in libido, and may find you even sexier now that you're a blossoming mother-to-be; in fact many couples report sex during pregnancy to be more intimate and bonding than usual. Other couples really enjoy the spontaneity of it, since there's no longer any pressure to avoid a pregnancy or to conceive one.

It takes two

However, don't be alarmed if your partner temporarily finds you less sexually attractive due to the changes in your body, or is concerned about hurting the baby during intercourse and wants to avoid it for that reason. He or she may also feel frustrated or neglected if your desire for sex has drastically diminished. In all cases, it's crucial that you talk about these changes openly and honestly, in a respectful, safe and non-accusatory setting.

If it turns out that your sex drives are not matching up, remember that there are many other ways to give and receive pleasure which don't involve actual intercourse. Massage, cuddling, snuggling, hugging and spending quality time together doing activities you both enjoy are other great ways to show your love for each other, and all of these activities are likely to increase production of the relaxing hormone oxytocin (read more about this on page 46). Manual stimulation or oral sex are perfectly safe during pregnancy (although you must never allow air to be blown into your vagina, as this can potentially cause an air embolism). Orgasm will not hurt the pregnancy, but it will cause uterine contractions – which are brief and harmless, but more noticeable when you're pregnant. And speaking of orgasms during pregnancy... don't be surprised if they're larger too – just like everything else.

Finding your groove

One thing is for certain – as your pregnancy progresses, your growing belly starts to make things a bit more logistically challenging. From the second trimester on, you should try to avoid positions which place weight directly on your belly. You might find yourself more comfortable on top, or making love in a side-lying position or from behind while standing. You can lean over and use the bed or the back of the couch as a prop, or get on your hands and knees (which has the added advantage of helping to relieve lower back pain as well), or sit in his lap. The sky's the limit, so long as you feel comfortable.

Anal sex is also fine during pregnancy, but all of the usual hygiene precautions are even more important in order to avoid an infection that could potentially spread to the baby. Vaginal intercourse should never be performed after anal intercourse without both partners thoroughly washing their genitals with soap and water, and changing the condom (if you used one). The same applies to sex toys.

Because your cervix is more sensitive and bleeds more easily during pregnancy, you might notice some light spotting after vaginal intercourse. This is caused by mechanical bruising of the cervix during penetration, and it may take up to 24 hours for the spotting to appear, but rest assured that this is very common after intercourse. As long as it's light (usually red or brown) and stops after another day or so, it's a normal response to intercourse. However, if the bleeding continues or worsens, or if you start to notice any regular or painful contractions, call your healthcare provider immediately.

> Felt totally hot today, and I'm not talking about the weather! #sexymum

Condensed idea
Your sexuality is bound to change during pregnancy, but sex is healthy and normal, and a great way to unwind

15 When things go wrong

Unfortunately 10–20 per cent of all confirmed pregnancies are lost, and still more may end before a woman even misses her period. This may be Mother Nature's way of ensuring that only healthy babies are born. Even so, a miscarriage can be very distressing.

Causes of miscarriage

When a miscarriage happens, women often ask 'Why? What caused this? What did I do wrong?' While there are no easy answers, miscarriages usually happen because there is some kind of problem with the developing embryo, and most pregnancy losses occur in the first trimester. Abnormalities with the number or structure of the chromosomes are very common (comprising 50–75 per cent of all miscarriages), which implies that there was a defect with either the egg or the sperm before fertilization even occurred. This also explains why older women experience miscarriage more frequently, as older eggs and sperm tend to have more defects. However, even if a perfect egg and sperm have found each other, problems can still arise with implantation or the formation of the placenta or baby. Think of all of the crucial developmental steps discussed on pages 16–19; if even one of those steps goes wrong or happens out of sequence, the baby's formation is affected and the body's answer is to miscarry.

Of course, there are other reasons for miscarriage. Conditions such as diabetes or thyroid disorders may cause miscarriage if left uncontrolled; with treatment, however, they are unlikely to cause any problems during pregnancy. Autoimmune conditions such as lupus have also been associated with higher rates of miscarriage. Other causes include exposure to toxins and chemicals, drug use (especially cocaine), infection and physical injury, such as a car accident. Even so, in the majority of cases, no cause is ever positively identified.

A brighter future

Surprisingly, if you've only had one miscarriage, your chance of having another successful pregnancy is just as good as if you've never been pregnant before. Even after two miscarriages, your chance of carrying a pregnancy to term is only slightly less than a woman who has never miscarried. However, after two miscarriages in a row, you might want to get yourself checked out to see if there's some kind of underlying cause, and after three in a row, it's imperative to do so. But be comforted: most women who have one (or even two) miscarriages are able to carry the next pregnancy to term without treatment.

Medical care

Contrary to popular belief, there is nothing you can do to prevent a miscarriage. Bed rest or avoiding physical exertion won't prevent one – nor will exercise or sex cause one. However, once you've been diagnosed with a miscarriage, treatment options vary. If you're already showing signs of impending miscarriage (bleeding and cramping), you and your doctor may decide on a 'watchful waiting' approach, meaning that you'll go home and wait for the miscarriage to occur, without any medical intervention. In

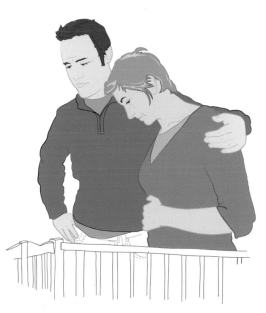

Warning signs of miscarriage

It is possible to experience miscarriage warning signs and not actually miscarry. However, when any of the following warning signs occur, the situation is called a 'threatened miscarriage' and requires attention. If you notice any of these signs, call your doctor immediately:

- Bleeding
- Cramping (anywhere from mild to intense)
- Spotting or staining even without any cramping or pain
- Fever
- Chills
- Foul-smelling vaginal discharge or pus
- Abdominal pain

most miscarriages, the body is able to spontaneously shed the products of conception without any extra help or intervention. However, sometimes there are no outward signs and a woman may miscarry without realizing it (this is called a 'missed abortion' in medical-speak). When this happens, the fact that a miscarriage has occurred is usually discovered during an ultrasound scan, when the sonographer is unable to detect a heartbeat. Given enough time – sometimes weeks – the body will often complete the miscarriage. However, in this situation a doctor may suggest other options to bring the situation to a close more quickly, such as performing a vacuum aspiration or an ERPC (evacuation of retained products of conception) to empty the uterus. If faced with this situation, it is fine to choose to wait or to opt for a procedure that will allow you more control over the ending of the miscarriage, as long as you are not showing any signs of infection (such as temperature, chills or muscle aches). Talk to your doctor about all of your options before making a decision, so that you feel confident about the medical management of the miscarriage. Regardless of how your miscarriage is treated, your doctor will want to see you one to two weeks afterwards, to confirm that the miscarriage is complete and that you are healthy.

Healing

When a woman miscarries, she mourns not only for the lost child, but also for the loss of a future that will no longer happen – all her parenting dreams and aspirations, and her hopes for that child. If you miscarry, you might find that even though you hadn't had a chance to meet your baby yet, she was very real to you. Your grief is just as real as it would be if you lost a beloved friend or family member, and you may go through the five stages of grief: denial, anger, bargaining, depression and acceptance.

Try to focus on the fact that most miscarriages occur for a reason and that nothing you did caused your own to happen. It's normal to feel sadness and loss, but sometimes women feel unjustified guilt, so tell yourself that this was not your fault; this was something beyond your control and there is nothing you could have done to prevent it. Reach out to your support network, and don't be shy about telling them what has happened. Miscarriage is not a taboo subject – and in sharing the news, you might discover a sisterhood of women who've gone through the same thing, and who are very likely to have gone on to have successful pregnancies afterwards. Lean on your partner and recognize that he or she is grieving too. And take your time – even though your body might be capable of another pregnancy with the very next cycle, you might not be ready. Listen to your heart and give it the time it needs as well.

Condensed idea
While surprisingly common, a miscarriage is still a very real and difficult loss

16 Location, location, location

These days, deciding where, how and with whom you want to give birth takes some thought. Although there are many options to suit your desires, budget and philosophy – the choices can be a little overwhelming at times. This chapter might help broaden your horizons.

Who's in charge?

The majority of doctors involved in delivering babies today are obstetricians: highly trained specialists in looking after pregnant women and their babies. However, other doctors who specialize in providing care to all members of the family (family or general practitioners) also receive obstetrical training during their residency and often provide some antenatal care. Caesarean sections are carried out by obstetricians with a team of medical staff.

A midwife is a skilled practitioner who specializes in normal pregnancy and vaginal birth, but not caesareans. Midwives often begin their careers as general nurses, then undertake additional training in midwifery. They generally care for healthy, low-risk pregnancies, but can also manage complications and some high-risk pregnancies, in collaboration with obstetricians. In the UK, midwives deliver 60 per cent of all babies born vaginally and they are the standard of care for healthy, low-risk pregnancies, both at home and in hospitals.

> Cosy home or high-spec hospital? Really can't decide where to have the little one. #toomuchchoice

Only you can decide

Before trying to make sense of the options, take some time to figure out what's important to you. Here are a few questions to think about:

- How important is having a natural birth to you?
- How important is having pain medication readily available to you?
- What feels best for you: foregoing some personal freedom in order to ensure that all technology is available should you need it, or maintaining your freedom in order to avoid unnecessary interventions?
- How do you picture your birth unfolding?
- Is it important to you that your care provider is a big part of your support team during labour?
- How important is being in a familiar, home-like environment to you?
- How important is continuity of care?

Worldwide, 60–80 per cent of babies are delivered by midwives, but in some countries, such as the USA, the majority of women receive all their care during pregnancy and labour from an obstetrician.

In terms of philosophy and approach, doctors tend to follow the medical model of care. They are trained to find and treat problems that arise in pregnancy, labour, delivery and after the birth, and their approach tends to result in a more controlled care. In contrast, midwives view pregnancy, labour and birth as a normal, physiological process that is inherently healthy. Rather than looking for pathology, they tend to trust the body, resulting in fewer routine interventions and more 'watchful waiting'.

Try to find a healthcare provider who shares and supports your views. The more comfortable you feel with your provider, the better your chance of having the type of experience you're looking for (being mindful that birth is not something you can control, so you will need to be flexible).

Home or hospital?

When thinking about the type of birth you'd like to have, it's important to think about the location that can best facilitate this experience. By far the most common location is the hospital. The advantage to giving birth here is that you will have all of modern medicine at your disposal. Should anything go wrong, an operating room is just down the hall. Your baby will be monitored closely throughout your labour, and a team of providers is available if needed, including an anaesthetist if you would like an epidural, and a paediatrician to care for the baby should any problems arise. The disadvantage of a hospital is that it can be very inflexible, unable to deviate from its policies and procedures, and there are other factors at play that can affect your birthing experience, such as staff coming and going, a busy ward, and restrictions on eating or drinking, freedom of movement, and visitors. In a hospital, you have to play by hospital rules, and sometimes this can lead to procedures or interventions which you were hoping to avoid.

The other end of the spectrum (and the least commonly taken option) is giving birth at home, usually with a midwife in attendance. The main advantages of delivering at home are total privacy, great flexibility and the security that stems from being in a familiar place. There are no rules except your own. Your body is allowed to labour and birth at its own pace, usually without any intervention, under the watchful eye of a midwife. However, choosing this setting brings with it many responsibilities, such as preparing your home for labour, cleaning up afterwards, and finding a healthcare provider willing to attend you at home. In the event of complications, you would probably need to be transferred to a hospital, and this can cost valuable minutes in an emergency situation.

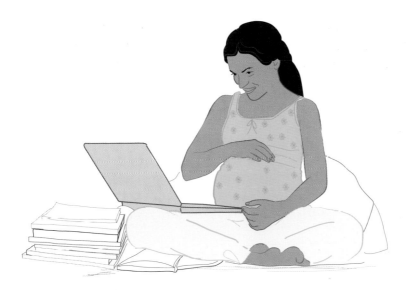

The final setting for birth is a birth centre – either attached to a hospital, or independent (i.e. in a separate building) which provides a nice middle ground if you don't want the confinement of a hospital or the responsibility of delivering in your home. Like hospitals, birth centres have policies and procedures in place which they adhere to, but they are generally designed for more flexibility and usually screen women so that only low-risk pregnancies can proceed there. Freedom of movement, the option to have a water-birth, the chance of fewer interventions and the more home-like environment are some of the many advantages to delivering in a birth centre. However, in an independent birth centre, you may still be many miles from a hospital and its technology – even an epidural is not an option. On the other hand, it may be the idea of a guided but natural birth that is a birth centre's biggest appeal.

Condensed idea
Do your research – make sure you get the type of care and location that you really want

Even just half a century ago, our ability to test the foetus was virtually non-existent. These days, though, we can do everything from ultrasounds to umbilical cord blood sampling, but deciding which tests to do – and even whether to do them – can still be tricky.

What are genetic tests?

Genetic tests offer you a way of either calculating the risk (probability) of certain genetic disorders, or directly taking material from the foetus to find out the actual chromosomal make-up of your child. Several genetic screening tests are done as part of your initial blood work, such as checking to see if you are a carrier for thalassaemia or sickle cell disease. Further tests are also occasionally done for inherited diseases, such as Tay-Sachs, which is present in people of certain ethnic groups. Additional screening tests, available at the end of the first trimester or in the second trimester, check for the risk of three specific disorders: Down's syndrome, Trisomy 18 and neural tube defects.

Screening tests

Screening tests are always non-invasive, meaning that they don't actually test the foetus directly. Instead, they test your blood for specific markers that can indicate an increased risk that your baby has the disease in question. In other words, they don't give you a yes or no answer – they simply calculate the chances of your baby having the disease, and indicate if further testing is needed. Since they're non-invasive, they don't actually pose any risks for your baby; they simply involve drawing a little blood from you.

The most common genetic screening tests in pregnancy check for the risk of Down's Syndrome and Trisomy 18, a similar condition. In the UK, women are screened between weeks 10 and 14 in two ways: through a blood test that estimates the woman's likely risk of carrying a baby with a genetic disorder, and via an ultrasound scan (the 'nuchal scan') that measures the amount of fluid under the skin of the baby's neck. The combination of information gained from these two screening tests, together with information on the woman's age, weight, family origin and health history, enables doctors to work out the risk of the baby having a genetic disorder. If you have these tests and are deemed to be at a raised level of risk, your doctors will suggest further, diagnostic tests.

Informed consent

Informed consent is a medical and legal concept based on the idea that you are a participant in your health care, and are capable of making your own medical decisions when given sufficient information.

During the informed consent process, the risks and benefits of each test or treatment will be explained to you by your health provider, together with any alternatives. While some of the principles of informed consent don't necessarily apply to antenatal testing (there aren't really any risks to having your blood type checked, for example), you still have the right to decline any tests you don't want, so long as you fully understand the risks you're incurring by declining. In general, you can always change your mind as well, although be aware that some tests, such as first and second trimester genetic screening, can only be done during very specific windows of time.

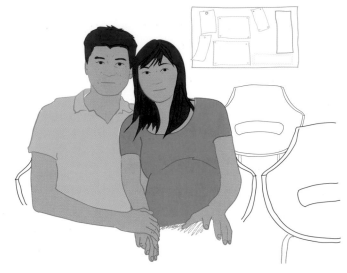

Diagnostic tests

Diagnostic tests are invasive, meaning that they sample fluids from the foetus or its environment directly, rather than examining markers in the mother's blood. Chorionic villus sampling (CVS) is usually done at 10–13 weeks in the UK, by taking a sample from the embryonic placenta through a small needle inserted either through the mother's abdomen or cervix under ultrasound guidance. Another test that may be carried out is amniocentesis, which is generally performed at 15–17 weeks. During this procedure doctors take a sample of amniotic fluid using a small needle and ultrasound, as for CVS.

Both CVS and amniocentesis have associated risks, particularly of miscarriage, which is why they are not performed unless other tests indicate that they may be necessary. For CVS, the risk is 0.5–1 per cent; the risk is slightly lower for amniocentesis (0.25–0.5 per cent). There are also risks of infection and loss of amniotic fluid if the small hole made in the membranes doesn't heal quickly, but this is rare. Other invasive techniques exist, such as percutaneous umbilical cord blood sampling (PUBS) and foetoscopy (placing a small camera inside the amniotic sac to view the foetus), but these tests are only done under very rare circumstances, because they contain much higher risks of miscarriage.

The advantage of having these tests is that they give you a definitive answer and tell you the exact chromosomal make-up of your child. If genetic disorders run in your family, you are likely to want to know whether your baby has developed a hereditary condition or not. These tests are often recommended for women over the age of 35, as the risk of Down's syndrome increases with the mother's age.

Why not test?

Worrying about whether your baby has an inherited disease or chromosomal defect is very frightening, and waiting for the results can be very stressful. However, it's worth remembering that the vast majority of screening tests come back indicating a low risk of a genetic disorder.

A screening test is not a guarantee, but a low risk result generally means that your baby has a low chance of having a genetic disorder. However, if the screening

> Worried about having an amnio but now so glad to know that everything's fine. #bigrelief

test indicates a higher risk (for example, 1 in 10), you will have to decide if you would like to proceed to invasive testing. In addition you'll also need to consider what you would do with the information. If you were to find out that your child has a genetic disease, for example, would you consider terminating the pregnancy? If you feel very strongly that you would never terminate a pregnancy, then what advantage do you gain from doing these tests? These questions are all incredibly personal, and will vary tremendously from one couple to the next.

Condensed idea
Genetic testing offers us a way to check for disorders, but some of the tests do carry risks

18 The growing bump

At last, you're showing. And that strange bubbly feeling that you may have thought was wind is actually the baby starting to move! She has all of her organs, but there's still a lot of growth and development going on in this trimester, so resting and eating well is still imperative.

Your baby at 13–28 weeks

Your baby already has all of her organs and structures in place, so the second trimester is all about adding important details. During this time, fine, downy hair, called lanugo, sprouts all over your baby, making her look a bit fuzzy (don't worry – by full term, nearly all of the lanugo has disappeared). In addition to this, small wispy eyelashes and eyebrows appear. By 22 weeks, your baby also begins to grow a small covering of hair on her scalp, which will continue to grow and thicken until full term, if she is destined to be born with a lot of hair on her head.

Your baby's motor development is also undergoing huge improvements during this time. At the very beginning of the second trimester, your baby can flex and extend her arms and legs, but as the weeks progress, these movements become much smoother, larger and stronger. Even though your baby has been moving for quite some time already, you'll finally be able to feel the movements yourself, an experience known as

> If I load up on broccoli and spinach now, will I have a toddler who eats her veg? #veggiemum

'quickening'. For first-time mums, quickening usually happens at 18–22 weeks; until that point, movements were always present, but you may have mistaken them for wind, bubbles or internal fluttering. If it's your second or third baby, it is more likely that you'll recognize the movements for what they are much sooner than you did the first time around, probably noticing them at around 16–18 weeks. By the end of the second trimester, the movements will be obvious to you (and you may even find they are sometimes a little painful) as your little one rolls, kicks, stretches, punches and dances around your womb.

Around 22–26 weeks, another delightful change begins: your baby starts to put on some weight. Up until this point, she's been incredibly lean, with muscles in place, but no subcutaneous fat at all under her nearly translucent skin. From 18 weeks onwards, the skin also becomes more opaque. A white, cheese-like substance called vernix caseosa also begins to form on the skin, which helps to protect your baby while underwater for nine months. At birth, and particularly if your baby is born prematurely, this cheesy, waxy substance can still be seen, especially in the skin creases. While many hospitals still routinely bathe babies shortly after birth, new research is uncovering the vernix's

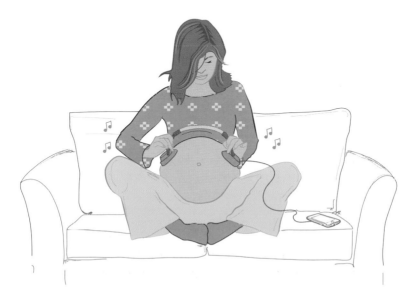

What they don't tell you...

Now that you're starting to look pregnant, there are some hidden perks (and hazards) to walking around in the world with an obvious bump:

- Perfect strangers may try to touch your belly. Your bump is not public property, though, so if this bothers you don't be shy about insisting on your personal space.
- People will (hopefully) start to offer up their seat to you on crowded trains or buses.
- Chivalrous individuals might offer to help carry your shopping out to your car or carry your bags for you – and if they do, the correct response is 'yes, please!' and 'thank you!'
- If you're still not showing much, don't be surprised if you hear a few comments (hopefully not to your face) about how you've been eating a few too many doughnuts lately.

amazing antimicrobial and immunity-boosting properties (which are nearly as strong as breast milk). So when the time comes for you to give birth to your baby, you may want to consider skipping the bath and simply rub the vernix into the baby's skin instead.

Your baby's lungs also continue their slow development throughout the second trimester. They're actually one of the last organs to mature, which means that often they are not ready to breathe on their own until late in the third trimester, when they produce a surfectant (a mix of fats and proteins) that will allow the lungs to expand during breathing. By 26 weeks, your baby's lungs will have matured sufficiently to give her a fighting chance at survival if she's born prematurely.

Your baby's senses

While it might seem like your baby is in a dark, protected environment, your baby's senses are actually more or less up and running by the second trimester, and reacting constantly to the many different stimuli she detects in the womb. She can hear by the end of the second trimester, and is rocked to sleep by the constant beat of your heart and the whoosh of your digestive system. She is alarmed by loud noises like sirens or shouting, and soothed by the sound of your voice speaking calmly, as well as familiar music and the voices of other family members. She might even respond to your voice with kicks or wiggles when you talk to her.

Your baby gains full touch awareness around 17–19 weeks. She will begin to explore this sense by stroking a hand or cheek or sucking on a finger, and by the third trimester, can actually feel your touch through your belly, which might explain why so many pregnant mums unconsciously rub their bellies. Your baby's sense of taste develops alongside her sense of smell, and amazingly, she can taste the foods you eat through her amniotic fluid, particularly strong flavours like garlic and curry, and will practice swallowing this fluid to prepare her for breast milk. She will prefer sweet flavours to sour or bitter ones, and once she's born she will have distinct taste preferences.

Even though vision is the last sense to develop (your baby sees her world in shades of black and white, and colour vision doesn't develop until approximately 2 months after she's born), she can see light filtering in through her closed eyelids, and will even turn away from bright lights in utero.

Condensed idea
By week 28, babies are so well developed that their chance of surviving premature birth is 90 per cent

19 Extra-special mums

Everyone would like to go through their pregnancy without a hitch, but often complications can arise. Whether your condition is common or potentially serious, the outcome is usually good and can make the journey more interesting.

Rh-negative mums

Doctors divide blood types into two main categories: Rhesus (Rh) positive or Rh negative. The majority of people are Rh positive, and for those who are Rh negative, it makes no difference at all – unless you are pregnant. During labour and birth, it's common for a small amount of the baby's blood to leak into the mum's blood system. If the mum is Rh negative but the baby is Rh positive, her body launches an immune response against the baby's blood, known as sensitization. When this happens, the mum's body forms antibodies designed to attack and destroy Rh positive blood in the same way that her immune system attacks and destroys foreign bacteria and germs. Unfortunately, once a woman is sensitized and these antibodies are created, she will have them for the rest of her life. In the past, this meant that Rh-negative women were able to have only one child safely – after the first pregnancy, her body would then attack all of her subsequent pregnancies, leading to severe foetal anaemia (known as haemolytic disease of the newborn) and sometimes foetal death.

Happily – and amazingly – in 1968 a treament was invented that can prevent sensitization. This treatment, known to mums as 'the anti-D injection', is given to the Rh negative mother at 28 weeks in the pregnancy and again after the baby is born if the baby's blood type is found to be positive. It's also injected after miscarriage, abortion or any invasive procedure that could cause blood mixing between mother and baby, such as an amniocentesis. Basically, the injection prevents the mother's body from recognizing the baby's blood and forming antibodies. If the father of the baby is Rh negative or the baby's blood type is Rh negative, anti-D is not needed after the delivery, but it will always be administered before the delivery as a standard part of prenatal care for Rh negative women.

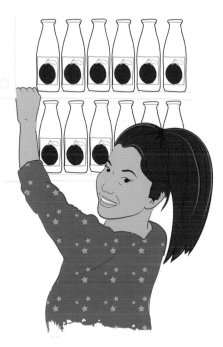

Prunes are a great way to boost iron stores and prevent that pregnant woman's bugbear, constipation

Anaemic mums

Babies are like iron sponges. It takes a lot of extra iron for the baby to form the haemoglobin in his system, and if you're not getting enough iron in your diet (or from supplementation), your baby is quite happy to suck the iron out of you – which can lead to maternal anaemia. For most women, this happens around 26 weeks, as this is the point when your blood volume has increased to its greatest amount, diluting the levels of iron (measured as haemoglobin) to its lowest point in the pregnancy. While anaemia is incredibly common, it can become quite dangerous if it gets too severe, particularly as you're bound to lose blood during birth (on average, women lose about 10 fl oz (300 ml) of blood in a vaginal delivery).

To combat this, your midwife or doctor will probably check your blood iron levels at the end of the second trimester, and if they are dropping, she will advise you on how much iron you should be taking to optimize your blood levels. Don't forget to eat your iron too (see page 78).

Iron, iron, iron!

Including more iron-rich foods in your diet is an excellent way to boost your iron levels during pregnancy.

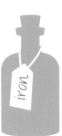

The foods on following list will help beef up your blood count, and don't forget the vitamin C – it helps your body absorb the iron, so take your iron supplements with orange juice or grapefruit juice, and add tomatoes to any nourishing beef or pork stews.

- Beans, beans and more beans!
- Meat, especially beef and pork
- Eggs (well-cooked)
- Dark green, leafy vegetables: greens, kale, chard and spinach
- Oatmeal
- Nuts, particularly cashews and almonds
- Whole wheat, shredded wheat and wheat germ
- Black treacle (delicious if added to porridge and oatmeal, poured over pancakes, or mixed into cakes or batter)
- Prunes! (your new best friend… a great source of iron, and a great way to help with iron-induced constipation!)

Diabetic mums

No one wants to hear that they have got gestational diabetes, but thankfully for most women who do develop it, the condition usually resolves itself after they have given birth. During pregnancy your body naturally becomes more insulin-resistant (insulin is the hormone needed to metabolize sugar), which means that there's more sugar floating around in your blood to help feed the baby. The combination of insulin resistance and an increase in blood sugar makes it much easier for pregnant women to become diabetic and, unfortunately, diabetes can cause several complications during pregnancy, such as pre-eclampsia and premature labour. Diabetes can also result in unusually large babies, who are more difficult to deliver due to their size. Such babies also have a much higher risk of shoulder dystocia, which occurs when the head is delivered but the shoulders get stuck.

I'm too sweet! Doc has me on a low-carb diet, but baby, you're worth it. #sugarfree

The good news is that with well-controlled sugar levels and careful monitoring, the chances are very good that these mums and babies will still have a healthy antenatal course. If you are diagnosed with gestational diabetes, you may even be able to control it with diet alone. You'll be placed on a low-carbohydrate, sugar-restricted diet, and will probably be asked to see a nutritionist or dietician.

Some women may need additional insulin or diabetic medicines, and all will receive additional monitoring throughout the pregnancy, such as ultrasounds and biophysical profiles in the third trimester (more on these on pages 112–15). Your labour may also be induced slightly early, as sometimes complications can arise if labour is allowed to occur on or after the due date.

Condensed idea
Good medical care can prevent many pregnancy 'complications' from turning into problems

(20) Aches and pains

By the start of the second trimester, energy usually returns, nausea retreats, and you start to get used to being pregnant. Your bump is still petite and manageable at this point, although the growing uterus can still give rise to some uncomfortable physical sensations.

Feeling the stretch

Two pieces of fibrous tissue (your round ligaments) anchor the top of the uterus to the tendons and other ligaments that surround your pubic bone and groin, and now that your uterus is starting to grow, these ligaments begin to pull and stretch, which can be quite painful at times. Imagine a large hot-air balloon filling with air and tugging on the ropes anchoring it to the ground – this is exactly what's happening as your uterus grows. Round ligament pain is often like a sharp stabbing feeling felt in the groin or lower abdomen radiating up both sides. It is usually worse when walking or moving, as this is when the ligaments have to work extra hard to keep the uterus in position and can sometimes become strained.

You may also feel this form of pain when rolling over, standing up quickly, laughing, sneezing or coughing. Don't worry, it's perfectly normal. Unfortunately, there's no cure for it besides giving birth, but you may find that changing position helps, as does yoga, which can help strengthen your core muscles. Wearing an abdominal support or brace may also ease the pain slightly. Moving slowly and taking your time when changing position may also give those over-stretched ligaments a bit of a break, while bending your legs slightly when coughing or laughing may avoid straining the ligaments. Rest assured that once your uterus is back to its normal size again, the pain disappears.

Sciatica

Like round ligament pain, this is a normal pregnancy discomfort most commonly felt from the second trimester onwards. It's caused most often by the baby's presenting part (usually the head) putting pressure on the sciatic nerve, which runs along the inner brim of the pelvis from the lower back, through the buttocks to the legs. When pressure is applied to this nerve, a sharp pain, tingling or numbness can be felt in the buttocks, hips, groin or thighs. Some women describe this feeling like lightning shooting down their legs. While sciatica can be excruciating at times, you can take comfort in the fact that it is not permanent – like round ligament pain, it will disappear shortly after the pregnancy. Until then, however, there's not much you can do about it. You can try shifting yourself into a different position when it strikes – sometimes leaning over on something or going down on hands and knees can help alleviate the pain. Some women have also experienced good results with massage, or by seeking out a good physical therapist or chiropractor.

> Pain so bad I woke up thinking I was in labour! Turned out to be leg cramp but oh so painful. #soembarrassed

A slower digestive system

While this might not be one of the complaints you usually hear about, constipation is actually incredibly common during pregnancy. There are three main culprits at work here. First of all, there is the pregnancy hormone progesterone, which slows down the movement of food through your intestinal tract so that your body can wring every last scrap of nutrition from it. Second, as your uterus begins to enlarge, it starts to displace the bowels, which makes moving food through your system even harder. And third, the increased amount of iron that you're eating doesn't help at all   iron is notorious for causing constipation.

Oh my aching legs!

Leg cramps are another very common symptom of pregnancy, and they can be excruciating. They usually hit you when you least expect it, causing you to wake up out of a deep sleep with a calf painfully knotted in spasm.

When leg cramps strike, try these home remedies:
- As soon as the cramp starts, try to stretch your calf – this will help ease it more quickly.
- Try increasing your calcium intake via more milk, cheese, yogurt and other dairy products, as sometimes low calcium can cause the cramping.
- Watch out for excess phosphorus, since this can also cause cramps – avoid processed foods, snacks and soft drinks.
- A magnesium supplement of 100–250 mg daily might also help, but check your prenatal vitamin – you may already be taking enough.

Luckily, there are a few remedies which do actually help. Load up on foods with lots of fibre in them, which is easy to do since these are all foods which are super healthy for you anyway – fresh fruits, vegetables and whole grains. Drink plenty of water, and give prunes and prune juice a whirl to see if this helps. When you do feel the urge to have a bowel movement, try to act on it promptly rather than holding it in. As with everything else, daily exercise will also make a difference. If absolutely necessary, a mild laxative might help, but clear its use with your midwife or doctor first. If none of these remedies make a difference and you still find yourself having a bowel movement every other day, this isn't dangerous and won't cause any harm to you or the baby.

Wind

Unfortunately, the increased levels of progesterone that are responsible for slowing down your intestinal tract also gives the food you ingest more time to ferment, which in turn creates more wind. In addition, because all of your muscles are being stretched and the baby is adding a great deal of pressure on top of it, you don't always have the same type of sphincter control you had before the pregnancy, which can lead to some embarrassing moments. Annoyingly, although perhaps reassuringly, this is all normal, and very common (although seldom mentioned). There's not much you can do

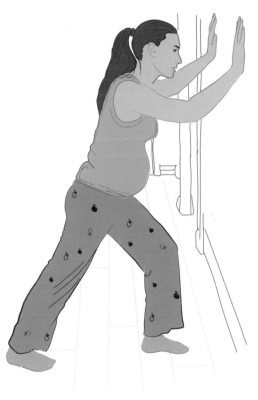

about it, but exercise will help (are you starting to notice a theme here yet?). As well as keeping yourself active, there are certain particularly gassy foods that you can avoid in your diet such as beans, broccoli, cauliflower, cabbage, dried fruits and fizzy drinks. Then hopefully those embarrassing moments will crop up a little less often!

Condensed idea
Aim to lessen the discomforts as much as you can, and start counting down the days until you deliver

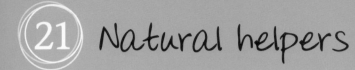

21 Natural helpers

A few natural remedies during pregnancy can sometimes make a huge difference to how you feel. Even if they don't completely relieve the discomfort, often the stress-relieving side effects are worth it in their own right, and they can be used at any time.

Yoga

Prenatal yoga is one of the best things you can do during pregnancy. Yoga is an excellent form of exercise, focusing in particular on the slow-twitch muscles (think endurance, which is what labour is all about) and building core strength. Because it's low-impact, you have a much lower chance of straining or injuring yourself, and all of the stretching exercises you do in yoga are fantastic for temporarily relieving sciatica, lower back pain and round ligament pain (see page 80). Yoga has been proven to help lower your heart rate and blood pressure, as well as boost your mood, concentration and memory.

> Breathing through a difficult pose yesterday was just like breathing through a contraction... I hope! #prenatalyoga

Yoga is also a unique way to strengthen your mind-body-spirit connection. Because the focus of yoga is on your breathing – and simply observing how your breath affects each part of your body – it's hard to worry about other things while you're doing yoga. The breath awareness keeps pulling you back to the present, and keeps you firmly grounded in your body. It also helps shut down signals from your sympathetic nervous system (responsible for fight or flight) and helps activate your parasympathetic nervous system (responsible for rest and relaxation) instead. Learning to calm yourself and focus on your breathing is also a fantastic tool for birth. The more you practice breathing awareness now, the easier it will be for you to use this skill in the face of pain during labour. You might also discover another hidden benefit to prenatal yoga – it puts you in a room full of other pregnant women!

A few extra goodies

Here are a few other natural things you can try during pregnancy to help relieve discomfort and prepare your body for birth:

- Red clover leaves and blossoms tea – this nourishes the entire reproductive system as a whole. It is also rich in trace minerals, calcium and magnesium.
- Rescue Remedy – a tincture based on the work of Edward Bach, a homeopath and pathologist of the 1930s, Rescue Remedy uses dilutions of flower essences to help promote emotional health. Some pregnant women find that a few drops taken 2–3 times a day in water can help stabilize their mood and bring a sense of peace and calm, and Rescue Remedy is safe to take during pregnancy.
- Homeopathy is a system of medicine that uses dilutions of plants and herbs to treat symptoms and emotional conditions. While homeopathy is generally considered safe during pregnancy since the remedies are so highly diluted, speak with your healthcare provider or homeopath before using any remedies.

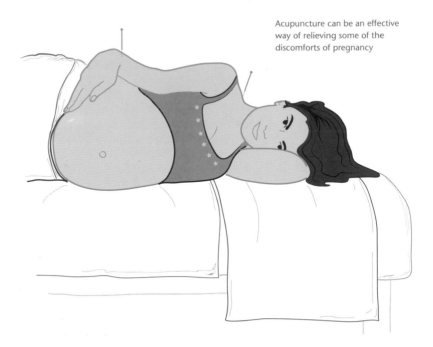

Acupuncture can be an effective way of relieving some of the discomforts of pregnancy

Acupuncture

Acupuncture is based on an ancient Chinese practice that promotes healing through the placement of very fine needles at specific body points in order to relieve tension and improve energy flow. While that sounds like it might be painful, most of the time you're so relaxed that you barely notice the needles being placed, and most sessions use shiatsu massage as part of the therapy. Today acupuncture can only be performed by a licensed practitioner who has trained and studied the practice for several years, and conforms to strict health standards with regards to hygiene and safety. Acupuncture is by no means a replacement for antenatal care, but it's a fantastic complementary therapy which is not only safe during pregnancy, but can sometimes relieve pregnancy symptoms which traditional Western medicine can't really help, such as morning sickness. It can also work magic on back and hip pain, help strengthen your immune system, and some studies have even shown that it can help relieve stress and effectively treat mild depression.

Sleep

This might sound really obvious, but getting enough sleep during pregnancy is one of the best ways to keep you and your baby healthy. Even though fatigue is a well-recognized pregnancy complaint, many women struggle to get enough sleep every day. In fact, pregnancy insomnia is a well-known and documented phenomenon, occurring most often in the late second and third trimester, when your large belly and active baby makes finding a comfortable position difficult, and your mind is occupied with concerns for the baby or the upcoming birth.

A few simple tricks might help make your nights more restful. First, get yourself a body pillow, or lots of extra pillows to tuck between your knees or under your hips at night. You can sleep in any position that's comfortable to you (sleeping on your belly won't hurt the baby in any way, although as your belly gets bigger this will gradually become uncomfortable). In the third trimester, it's important to avoid sleeping flat on your back, since this compresses the vena cava (the large vein which runs beneath your uterus and carries blood back to your heart), so be sure to prop your head up slightly, or put a pillow under your hip if you're on your back. Pick a regular bedtime, and try to stick to it no matter what. In the evenings, before you go to bed, try to unwind with an hour or two of relaxation beforehand, such as taking a bath, reading a book, listening to calming music or meditating (watching TV or a movie before bed is stimulating rather than relaxing, so try to avoid these activities right before you turn in for the night). Drinking a cup of warm milk with honey is another natural sleep aid (warming the milk releases the amino acid tryptophan, which makes us sleepy).

Condensed idea
There are many natural ways to boost your comfort and health during pregnancy

What's a birth plan?

Many people find that making a birth plan helps them prepare for the big day. However, labour is not something you can control, and it's important to remember that things may not go exactly as planned. Nevertheless, you may find the process helpful in itself.

It's all in the plan

A birth plan is a written document that spells out your preferences, hopes and deepest desires for your labour and birth. In deciding to write a birth plan, many couples find themselves thinking about their wishes for their birth in a more concrete way, and the act of writing a plan encourages researching different options and making decisions. Writing a birth plan can also bring you face to face with many of your deepest held beliefs about birth, as well as your fears and concerns, and force you to confront them and process them, which is all very valuable work.

> Birth plan: written! Birthing playlist: underway! My, what a productive week it's been. #2ndTri

The majority of birth plans focus on who will be present at the birth, the type of environment you're looking for, desires for pain medication (or desire that pain medication not be offered unless requested), labour support methods you'd like to use (position change, walking, birthing balls, aromatherapy, music etc.), interventions which you're hoping to avoid (or have), and your wishes for the baby in the immediate newborn period. There are plenty of birth plan templates available online to look

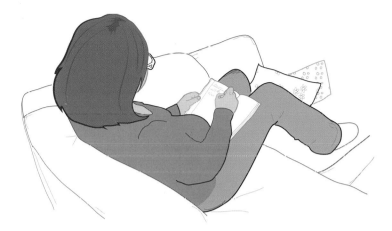

at – some templates even offer you the ability to check off what you'd like from a long list – but the best birth plans come from the heart and are written by you from scratch.

We looked earlier at how important it is to work out your expectations and preferences (see pages 64–67) in order to find the right care provider who could best support your desires; writing a birth plan is an extension of this. Many women find that in researching their options for their birth plan, they discover a lot more about the kind of birth they're hoping for, which can lead to some important and valuable conversations with your midwife or doctor. In some cases, it can also lead to either changing the setting of your birth in order to better align with your plan, or finding a different care provider whose philosophy better complements your own.

Go with the flow

Writing a birth plan can sometimes lead to unintended consequences. If you've put a lot of time and care into spelling out your wishes and desires for every stage of the labour, you might find yourself incredibly disappointed or angry if your plan isn't followed to the letter. Sometimes the baby doesn't give you a choice because she has her own ideas about how she's going to be born, or emergencies arise which require deviating

Hopes, wishes, desires

If you're still unsure about what should go in your birth plan, or what kind of birth philosophy you have, use the sentence stemming technique discussed in the text box in Chapter 3 (page 15) to come up with 7–10 endings for the following statements (and revisit Chapter 16, which also has a few ideas about your birth expectations) to start your thought process:

• When I think of myself in labour, I am…
• I realize that the things I can control in labour are…
• I realize that the things I can't control in labour are…
• When I am feeling vulnerable and uncertain, I am comforted by…
• I am hoping that my birth will be…
• The part of labour I am most looking forward to is…
• The part of labour I am least looking forward to is…
• When I envision myself giving birth, I see…
• The people in the room with me during my labour are…

from the plan entirely. You may even consciously decide to change your plan in the middle of labour as your birth unfolds, such as choosing to forego the pain relief you thought you needed because you're finding that you're able to cope with the contractions much better than you anticipated – or the opposite! Labour is completely unpredictable, and not something which you can control. The most important permission to give yourself during labour is the freedom to be flexible, along with a willingness to roll with the punches.

There are some birth educators who advise against a written birth plan. While incredibly individual, birth plans are generally asking for the same thing – the desire to be included in decision-making, the desire to be treated with respect and dignity, and the desire to have your preferences consulted throughout the birth. These are universal rights, which every couple is entitled to, and some people argue that you don't really need a written plan to help enforce this. Others suggest writing out your birth plan, and then symbolically ripping it up. The process of thinking about your hopes and preferences and the act of writing it down helps you clarify your desires, but the act of ripping it up gives you a sense of freedom and flexibility, and reminds you that you don't really need a plan spelling out every aspect of the labour in order to give birth. Birth is a natural process, after all, and you are quite capable of it even without any prior thought or attention.

Birth vision

It might be easier to think about a birth vision, rather than a birth plan. This is a subtle distinction, but it can make a big difference on the day itself. Birth plans can sometimes become too specific and tend to focus on the negatives (things you don't want rather than things you do), whereas a birth vision focuses more on the general goals and philosophies you'd like to keep in mind while in labour. It might be helpful to write down your birth vision in your pregnancy journal, or write it like a letter to yourself and to those who will be supporting you in labour. Once you've completed your vision, be sure to share it with everyone who will be present at your birth (including your midwife or doctor) so that they will know how best to support you during this incredible rite of passage.

Condensed idea
Work out a birth plan but be ready to let it go if the need arises

(23) The dream team

You're probably wondering about who should be there with you during the birth. Your partner will hopefully be first choice, but you may want others too. Putting together a good support team takes some thought, but the benefits are priceless when push comes to shove.

Good support is hard to find

Deciding on your labour support team is a very personal decision. Ideally, the people in the room with you when you give birth will be people that you are totally comfortable with, trust emphatically, find calming and relaxing, and who understand and support your birth vision, recognizing that this is your journey, not theirs. While that last bit might sound harsh, it's important to keep in mind that during labour you won't have any extra energy to give to anyone else. So whoever you choose should be your choice, and not pushed on you or taken for granted in any way (for example, your mother, sister or in-laws). It's also important to keep in mind that your support team will see aspects of you which they've most likely never seen before, so it's crucial that you don't feel shy or embarrassed in front of them, particularly with regard to all of the bodily fluids and processes involved.

Whomever you decide on, be sure to speak with them beforehand so that they're aware of their role and what you expect from them. Perhaps you want the bulk of your support to come from your partner, but would like your mother or friend there to help support him or her, You may like to designate someone to time the contractions, call the midwife, or keep you and your partner fed, and so on. No matter what their role, be sure to discuss your wishes with them well in advance of the labour, so that they can help support you. You might suggest that they read a few books about labour support to help prepare themselves, or attend a childbirth education class with you or on their own. It's also important to make sure they will be available from the 37th week of the pregnancy onwards. Attending a birth is always an honour and a privilege, and it's important that your support team knows this and treats the event with respect.

Labour etiquette

Once you've decided who will be in the room with you, it might help to talk a little bit about labour etiquette beforehand. Go through the guidelines below with your support team, and feel free to add any others which you think are appropriate:

- Silence is golden – if the people around you during labour aren't speaking to you directly, ask them to refrain from other conversations, as talking about their weekend plans (for example) will pull the energy away from you, and make it harder for you to concentrate and relax.
- Keep mobile phone use to a minimum – your other friends and relatives don't need a minute-by-minute text update. If you like, you can designate a 'point-person' to send updates to, and then he or she can update the rest of the family on your behalf.
- Take a position on photography, depending on how important privacy is to you. You can ask that no photos be taken, or designate a single photographer.
- Suggest that your team might like to read a labour-support book before the great event. *The Birth Partner* by Penny Simkin is a great place to start.

The doula difference

A doula (pronounced doo-la) is an experienced labour support person who is there to offer continuous physical, emotional and practical support to you during the labour and birth. Doulas are also available in the immediate postnatal period (although many tend to specialize in either birth or postnatal). She will generally come to your house at the very start of labour, and will stay with you until a few hours after the birth, helping you breathe, relax, cope with your contractions or navigate the hospital system – whatever you find you need. While most doulas are trained and certified these days, they provide a support role only, and are not medically licensed to diagnose or treat any aspect of your labour (that's what your midwife or doctor is for). However, since a doula will have attended many other births, she can usually provide an invaluable perspective based on her experience, and is excellent at helping to support and advocate for you, particularly in a hospital setting.

> So I think I'll need two other people with me at the birth – one to support me, and one to support Dan when he passes out. #birthplan

Many remarkable studies have been done on doulas which have convincingly demonstrated that having a designated labour support person can help shorten your labour, improve your chances of delivering naturally and improve outcomes for both you and your baby. Having an experienced support person there can not only help reassure you, but also your partner, who is likely going through his or her own apprehensions. A doula will take some of the pressure off your partner, and give him or her the freedom they need to go through their own birth journey and transition as well. While you might be wondering at the need (and expense) of an extra labour support person, many women find their doula to be worth every penny.

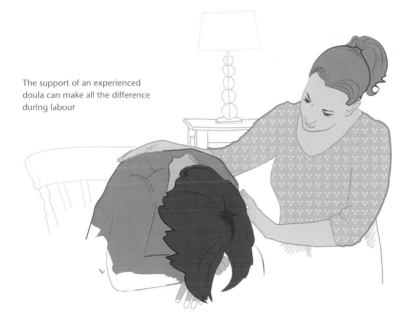

The support of an experienced doula can make all the difference during labour

Anyone else?

When you arrive at the hospital, you will be assigned to a labour and delivery nurse, or to a midwife, who will be spending most of the next few hours with you, and is responsible for monitoring the progress of your labour and making sure that both you and the baby are doing well. She will also be working closely with whoever will be doing the delivery, if she's not doing it herself. You may also have an anaesthetist present if you opt for an epidural or have a caesarean section. If necessary, a paediatrician or neonatologist may also be present at the birth to check the baby or perform resuscitation as needed.

Condensed idea
Choose your support team carefully, and don't let anyone else make the decision for you

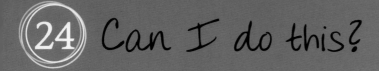

(24) Can I do this?

As the delivery date draws nearer, you may start asking yourself: 'will I be any good at this whole parenting thing?' In some ways, worry is how your subconscious prepares you for the big things in life, and you probably have much less to worry about than you think.

Relax, you're doing well

Pregnancy can be a really anxiety-inducing time in your life. Your body is going through huge changes, many things seem out of your control (like those stretch marks which just magically appeared last week, despite your daily moisturizing routine), and it's hard to know what's going to come next. It's normal to worry about whether you're eating right, whether your baby will be normal and healthy, or whether you'll go into labour early and have to deal with prematurity. That's plenty to keep you up at night, so it's no wonder pregnant women often experience insomnia!

However, try your best to breathe a big sigh of relief. The majority of babies (96 per cent) are born healthy, without birth defects. So long as you're eating well, taking your prenatal vitamins and avoiding the big no-no's (smoking, alcohol, drugs), you're probably on track to produce a perfectly healthy, normal baby. Additionally, thanks to genetic testing and scans, many problems are discovered before you actually give birth, and remarkably, some of them are actually treatable while you're still pregnant. So even if there is something unusual going on, there are steps that can be taken to prepare for the delivery, such as moving to a different hospital with a better neonatal intensive care unit, or having paediatrician specialists on hand to ensure that your baby gets the optimal care he needs.

Common concerns

The other big concerns which start to crop up now (but generally intensify in the third trimester, as the due date begins to loom on the horizon) are worries about the birth itself. You might find yourself thinking: will I be able to push my baby out? What will labour feel like? Will I be able to handle the pain? What if I poo on my midwife? What if my private parts never recover? What if I need a caesarean?

These fears are incredibly common – speak to a few other pregnant friends about their worries, and similar concerns are bound to be voiced by everyone you talk with. And it's hard to know what labour will be like; it's a great unknown, a mystery and a rite of passage all at the same time, and it will be different for every single person who goes through it. Naturally, because it's something you've never done before, you're going to wonder if you can do it or not, and you won't know for sure until the moment comes, so it doesn't help to worry about it beforehand. Trust is a good word to think about in labour – surrender yourself up to your labour,

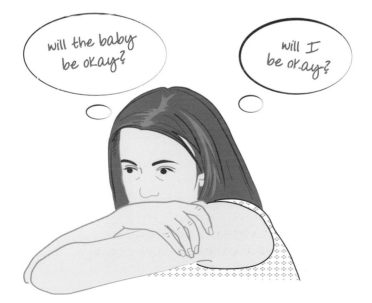

The power of positive thought

Hypnobirthing is a childbirth education method which prepares women for natural labour through the use of hypnosis. Part of their preparation before the birth includes the use of pregnancy affirmations, which helps programme your psyche on its deepest level. Feel free to write your own affirmations, or revise the ones below (adapted from *Hypnobirthing: A Celebration of Life* by Marie Mongan) so they reflect your deepest beliefs, and then practise saying these to yourself several times a day, like a mantra.

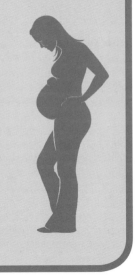

- I will carry my baby to term.
- I will have a healthy baby and be healthy myself.
- I put all fear aside as I prepare for the birth of my baby.
- I trust my body, and I follow its lead.
- I am focused on a smooth, easy birth.
- My mind is relaxed; my body is relaxed.
- I feel confident; I feel safe; I feel secure.
- I will yield to the power of my body.
- I am prepared to meet whatever turn my labour takes.

to the wisdom of your body, and trust that your body is absolutely 100 per cent perfectly designed to give birth, and to heal afterwards. Labour is not like an exam you have to pass – there is no right or wrong way to give birth. It probably won't go at all like you've planned, but the chances are that whatever labour brings, you will be able to handle it. Remember too that you'll have a team of supporters and medical practitioners watching out for you and your baby, should anything even start to go off the rails.

As to the other concerns, when you begin to push, it's true that many women push out a small amount of stool before the baby, and your

> None of my terrors turned out to be true. Trust me, our bodies are more capable than we think #newmum

practitioner will take it as a good sign when they see this – it means that you're pushing effectively! No one in the labour room will be horrified by this (they've seen it all a thousand times before), so feel free to leave your embarrassment along with your coat at the door. As for your poor nether regions, you might be comforted to know that your vagina is one of the most forgiving parts of your body, and thanks to the bountiful blood flow to the area, healing usually occurs very quickly. While most women do tear a bit, the vast majority are completely healed and back on their feet in six weeks or less; most of the time you can't even see a scar afterwards.

Becoming a mother

The thought of becoming a parent and taking on the responsibility of caring for and raising a child is certainly sobering, but the good news is that your ability to parent grows as your child does. It's a learned skill, and a dynamic transition. In the beginning, as you're coping with sleep deprivation and taking care of a small baby with constant needs, parenting style is the last thing you're thinking of, but you'll learn from your child and gradually gain confidence. You won't know what kind of parent you are (or want to be) at this stage – only experience can teach you that, so for now, mothering and nurturing yourself is the best way to mother and nurture your baby.

Condensed idea
Worrying is a normal part of pregnancy, but complications are rare, so focus on the positives

(25) Big and slow

Towards the end of the second trimester, the physical reality of the pregnancy begins to set in as you find yourself bigger and slower than you've ever been before. While this can be a bit disconcerting, you'll be surprised by how quickly you'll adapt to your new body.

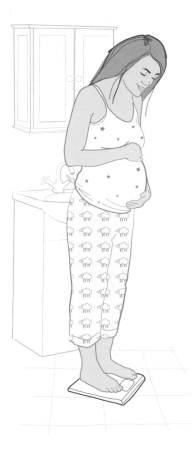

Living large

Let's face it, being pregnant is all about the burgeoning belly, and it's really starting to make its presence felt now. As more and more weight is carried at your front, your lower back begins to compensate by curving more than normal (known as lordosis), which begins to produce the classic pregnancy waddle. This also throws off your centre of gravity a great deal, which means that you can no longer spring out of your chair, whizz round tight corners or manoeuvre in close quarters. Getting around gradually starts to take longer and longer as you sometimes begin to feel like a truck with a 'wide load' sign on the back.

Your hips also experience change during pregnancy. Due to the hormone relaxin, which is produced in larger quantities as your pregnancy progresses, all your ligaments and tendons begin to relax and stretch, giving your joints – and especially your hips – much more mobility than they usually have. This can give you a strangely loose feeling in your pelvis, making you feel quite disjointed. Sometimes wearing a pregnancy support belt or girdle can help combat this sensation.

Big is beautiful

The extra kilos gained in pregnancy may be difficult, especially for those who have struggled with their weight or body image before, but it's worth remembering that it's usually temporary and it's your body's way of protecting the baby that you're growing. For women who have struggled to conceive, the weight gain and belly can be a wonderful reminder of success. For those who normally have small breasts and have often wondered what it

> Can't believe I forgot my own wedding anniversary! OMG, where has my mind gone?!? #babybrain

would be like to experience a C-cup, this is the time to enjoy temporary largesse. And for women who may have spent years worrying about their belly, now's the time to embrace it! The important thing to remember is that your body is doing what it needs to in order to grow and carry a life. Try to eat a balanced diet and stay active, but don't beat yourself up if pregnancy cravings make an occasional ice-cream sandwich seem like a paramount need.

How much weight will I gain?

Weight gain is always an area of concern. You may never have weighed this much before, and might feel slightly alarmed by your rapid weight gain, especially during the third trimester. Just remember that weight gain is necessary to ensure a healthy pregnancy and birth, and to help

Embrace your pregnant body!

You might have been raised to think that less is more, but consider some of the many advantages to being more substantial:

- Getting a seat on the bus or train is suddenly much easier.
- If you have to sit for a long time on a hard seat, it's not such a hardship any more.
- You can now wear all of the cleavage-revealing clothes that never worked on you before.
- Maternity clothes (which have lots of growing room) may be among the most comfortable wardrobe items you'll ever wear!
- Extra padding keeps you warmer in the winter – kiss those extra cardigans goodbye!
- Curves are more cuddly.

support your baby afterwards once you're breastfeeding. Weight gain guidelines are based on studies which have demonstrated the optimal amount needed to produce a healthy, full-term baby with a normal birth weight (usually 2.8–3.5 kg/6–7½ lb). At the start of your antenatal care, your healthcare provider will probably check your BMI (body mass index) and advise you on how much weight you should ideally gain. In general, women with a low BMI are advised to gain about 16 kg (35 lb) throughout the pregnancy; those with a normal BMI are advised to gain roughly 13.5 kg (30 lb); and those overweight are advised to gain 11 kg (25 lb) or less.

In the first trimester, weight gain is usually very minimal, perhaps 1–2 kg (2–5 lb) total for the entire trimester. After that, most women find themselves gaining 0.2–0.5 kg (½–1 lb) a week for the rest of the pregnancy. Weight loss during pregnancy is never recommended, although it may inadvertently happen in the first trimester. Your body (and baby) needs those extra pounds! Try not to stress too much about how much you're gaining; most women have a built-in super-diet waiting for them on the other side of labour, known as breastfeeding.

Baby brain

Around this time in the pregnancy, another strange phenomenon often develops known as 'baby brain', where you become much more forgetful or scatter-brained than normal. While some experts claim it's all a myth, recent studies have suggested that the hormonal changes in the pregnancy do in fact affect memory and your ability to focus.

You might find yourself unable to remember the names of people you know incredibly well, or forget items or people you were just talking about. Baby brain also makes it very hard to pay attention or follow through on routine tasks. Many women find themselves starting one task, getting distracted by something else, and then completely forgetting that they had even started the first task – until they stumble upon it again 10 minutes later.

Trust us: you're not going crazy! The phenomenon of 'baby brain' is a very common occurrence during pregnancy (and up to one year after you have the baby, too) and some researchers even suggest that it serves a purpose. In making women more easily distracted, a lack of complete concentration helps ensure that a woman will be able to put down whatever she's doing and tend to her baby when needed, rather than continuing her current task.

Condensed idea
Bumps are meant to get bigger and bigger, and bigger!

26 Early babies

While figures for premature labour are on the rise, half of all women who experience it still manage to carry their babies to term. But even if it does lead to premature birth, babies born as early as 28 weeks have a 90 per cent chance of survival without impairments.

Premature contractions

'Premature labour' is the experience of premature contractions that cause cervical dilation, well before labour is due. It is possible to have premature contractions that don't actually dilate your cervix and kick you into labour, although telling the difference can sometimes be tricky. A new test known as the foetal fibronectin test can now help distinguish between the two. This test is performed between weeks 23–34 of the pregnancy if you have any contractions during that time, by taking a swab of vaginal secretions. If the amniotic sac has begun to separate from the uterine wall, the swab will show signs of a substance known as foetal fibronectin – you can think of it as a glue holding the baby within the uterus – and normally it isn't present in the vagina unless birth is imminent. If foetal fibrinectin is detected, the risk of going into labour in the next two weeks is slightly increased. If the test comes back negative, you have a 96 per cent chance of not going into labour in the next two weeks. As this result is quite accurate, a negative test is incredibly reassuring.

In addition to a foetal fibronectin test (or sometimes in lieu of this test), you will be placed on an electronic foetal monitor to assess the duration and frequency of your contractions, and also to confirm that your baby is doing just fine. Your urine will most likely be checked for a urinary tract infection, and your vaginal secretions may also be examined for infection as well. Your doctor may also examine your cervix to see if there is dilation; if so, you'll probably be checked again a few hours later to see if the dilation is increasing. Some healthcare providers also use vaginal ultrasound to evaluate the length and thickness of the cervix – when you're in labour, the cervix begins to thin and dilate, and this is visible on ultrasound. Depending on what's going on, your treatment options will be tailored to the gestational age of your baby and how quickly the labour is progressing.

Premature labour warning signs

While not all premature contractions lead to premature birth, you should be on the look out for any of the signs below, and notify your doctor immediately if any of these occur:

- Regular contractions – this is defined as 5 or more contractions in an hour, or contractions every 10–15 minutes.
- Any dribbling or leaking of fluid – this is sometimes just a few drops rather than a huge gush; if you're not sure whether your waters have broken, let your healthcare provider know so he or she can assess you.
- Any bleeding or spotting, particularly if it's heavy and fresh (bright red as opposed to brown or pink).
- Decreased foetal movement – while this is not really a sign of premature labour, it's always an ominous sign and should prompt swift assessment in order to confirm that the baby is doing well (see pages 112–15 to find out more about how to count and assess normal foetal movement).

Premature causes

The causes of premature birth are still not fully understood. It is thought that there are four main pathways which can lead to early activation of labour: an early trigger arising from the baby's endocrine (hormonal) system, uterine overdistension (where the uterus stretches too much – this helps explain why twins are usually born premature), decidual bleeding (bleeding occurring between the placenta and the uterine wall), and intrauterine inflammation and/or infection. Urinary tract infections, kidney infections and even gingivitis (gum disease) have also been implicated in increasing the risk of premature contractions. Dehydration can increase the likelihood of premature contractions (although not necessarily premature labour), and your age and ethnicity also play a role. While the reason behind this is not fully understood, it's been observed that women at the extreme ends of childbearing (younger than 18 years old, and older than 35) have much higher rates of premature labour, as do women of African descent (as opposed to Caucasian, Asian or Hispanic).

> The doc says that the contractions look pretty regular, and I'm only 32 weeks pregnant. Yikes! We're not ready! And neither is Peanut! #tooearlytobemum

Treatment

Usually the first line of treatment for premature contractions is IV hydration (being given fluid via a drip), because dehydration is often the culprit, and hydration alone is often enough to put an end to them. However, if contractions continue and dilation occurs despite the hydration, or if your waters have broken or you have a positive foetal fibrinectin test, other medicines may be used to try to slow down the labour. Generally, once premature labour is diagnosed, you will be admitted to hospital. If an infection is suspected, this will be treated

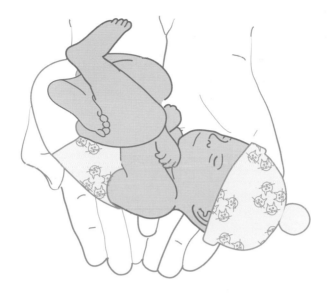

too, usually with a course of antibiotics. Most women with premature contractions are also given a course of steroids (either dexamethasone or betamethasone) to help prepare the baby's lungs in anticipation of a premature birth. Studies have shown that premature babies who have received steroids before birth require less assisted ventilation than babies who didn't, and generally have a much easier time adapting to life outside the womb.

If a premature delivery is anticipated, a paediatric team will be on hand to help with the baby immediately after the delivery. For nearly all babies born less than 32 weeks of age, a stay in intensive care is often unavoidable. For late premature deliveries (34–36 weeks), babies will be very carefully monitored but may not require admission to intensive care, depending on their condition.

Condensed idea
Act immediately if you have any warning signs of premature delivery

(27) Third trimester baby

The third trimester is about putting the finishing touches to your baby's organs and parts, and growing. In fact, nearly two-thirds of your baby's final birth weight is acquired in the last four weeks of the pregnancy alone, as well as all kinds of other miraculous developments.

Your baby at 28 to 40 weeks

While all of the initial organ growth and development occurred in the first trimester and early second trimester, there are plenty of organs which still require time to mature, and a few final details that need to fall into place. Your baby's fingernails, for instance, have been growing from the first trimester, but they finally reach the fingertips by about 34 weeks. The hair on his head is becoming thicker and more lustrous, and the coating of vernix (the white waxy substance) protecting the baby's skin thickens as well. Around 31–32 weeks, the fine downy hair known as lanugo, which has been covering and protecting your baby's skin, begins to fall off, making him look much more human and much less like a little monkey. However, small patches of it may remain by the time he's born, especially on his back and arms, although it will eventually disappear altogether.

Around 28 weeks your baby cracks open his eyes for the very first time, and can now bat his beautiful set of eyelashes, which have just grown. By 30 weeks in the pregnancy he's able to open his eyes wide, and will keep them open for several hours throughout the day. By 33 weeks in the pregnancy, his pupils dilate, constrict and react to light, and he is now able to perceive light shining through your skin and into your womb, brightening his environment.

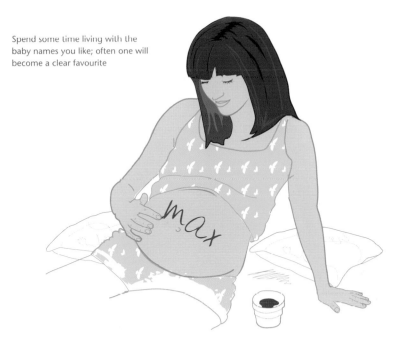

Spend some time living with the baby names you like; often one will become a clear favourite

Your baby's sex organs are also finishing their development. If you have a boy, his small testes begin to descend from his abdomen into the scrotum starting in the eighth month, and will usually complete their descent by the time he is full term. Occasionally, in around 3–5 per cent of cases, one or both testicles fail to descend by the time of birth, although in most cases, they complete their descent by four months of age (sometimes surgery is needed to help this process along if it doesn't happen on its own). In little girls, the labia are completely differentiated by the eighth month, and the labia majora usually grow to the point that they cover and enclose the clitoris and labia minora by full term.

By 36 weeks, the baby is about as long as he's going to get in the womb, and from here on nearly all of his growth is focused on weight rather than height. The skin is now completely opaque, and appears smoother; small rolls of subcutaneous fat begin to accumulate, making him finally look like the chubby baby you've probably been dreaming about. While the size of term babies varies greatly, by full term (37 weeks) they average 3.4 kg (7½ lb) in weight and 45 cm (18 in) in length.

What's in a name?

At this point in the pregnancy, you're probably starting to think a lot more seriously about what to call your little one after the birth. While some couples know the names of their future babies before they're even conceived, many couples still wait for several days after the birth before choosing a name. Here are a few tips and fun facts to keep in mind when deciding:

• Pick a name with staying power – sure, it might sound cute when he's a toddler, but imagine him introducing himself at a job interview… will it still be acceptable then?
• If you like a shortened version of a name (Bill for William, or Kate for Katherine), put the longer version on the birth certificate. You can always use the nickname, but your baby will have the option of the longer name as an adult.
• Bear in mind that spelling matters – choosing to spell a popular name in an unusual manner will certainly make your baby unique, but may cause headaches and confusion on documents, applications, and even the birth certificate (it's Jane Eyre, after all, not Jehyne Aiyre).
• Middle names can certainly be creative – and feel free to add as many as you like – but double check all of the initials to make sure they don't spell anything unwanted. (Arthur Samuel Smith? Chris P. Bacon, anyone?)
• Make a short list, then practise saying each of the names out loud, with middle and last names attached.
• Many parents decide to wait until the baby is born to see what he or she looks like before deciding on the final name.

Ready to breathe?

You'd think that one of the most important organs for survival would also be one of the first to develop, but in fact, your baby's lungs are one of the very last organs to come up to speed (although your baby starts practising his breathing well before the lungs are actually ready to function). Surfactant production begins around 26 weeks, and is usually complete by 38 weeks. Surfactant is a soap-like compound that allows the small air sacs

> Nearly there now. Doc says she'd be ready even if she arrived tomorrow. #justwaiting

(alveoli) of the lungs to expand with air rather than stick to each other – your baby needs an adequate supply in order to breathe air (rather than depending on you for his oxygen supply).

If for some reason your healthcare provider is considering an induction or caesarean before your due date, they may talk to you about performing an amniocentesis to check the L:S ratio before beginning the induction. This is a measurement of surfactant and lung maturity in your baby and it involves taking a very small sample of amniotic fluid for testing.

By 37 weeks gestation nearly every baby's lungs are mature, but in some cases they may be fully mature as early as 36 weeks, or as late as 38 weeks. As discussed earlier (see pages 104–107), if for some reason you're anticipating a premature delivery, you will also probably be given a course of steroids in order to help promote surfactant production in your baby and speed up the maturation process.

condensed idea
By 36 weeks, your baby is fully developed and all the growth is weight gain

Checking it out

Now that your baby is moving regularly, foetal movement becomes one of the most reliable ways to check on your baby's wellbeing. Other tests that can be carried out include monitoring the baby on a foetal heart monitor or imaging him with ultrasound scans.

Baby movement

When your baby is moving, you can breathe a big sigh of relief because it means that your baby is doing well. It's literally not possible for your baby to move too much – the more the better! In contrast, lack of normal foetal movement should be investigated immediately. Keep in mind, though, that each baby has his or her own pattern. By 28–30 weeks into the pregnancy, these patterns are usually well established. Some babies are very active, others more chilled out; some babies prefer to move at

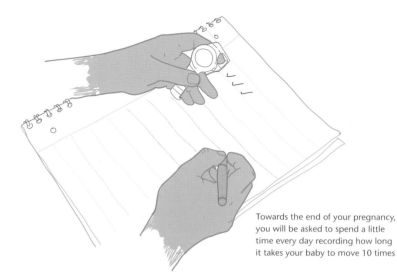

Towards the end of your pregnancy, you will be asked to spend a little time every day recording how long it takes your baby to move 10 times

Counting movements

Foetal movement counts, also known as 'foetal kick counts', are a very simple way for you to confirm that your baby is fine. There are many different ways to do this test, and your doctor or midwife will probably give you specific instructions, but in general, it involves timing how long it takes for your baby to make 10 movements on a daily basis. Women are usually asked to start counting movements at around 36 weeks in the pregnancy (although you may be asked to begin sooner than that). Here are a few tips to make this exercise easier:

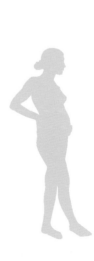

- Write down the time you start paying attention, then put a check on the paper every time you feel a movement. Stop counting when you reach 10, and write down the time again. Don't let yourself become distracted by other things.
- Every movement counts, no matter how big or small – kicks, twists, squirming, punching and bobbing are all fine, but hiccups don't count.
- In general, it should take between 30 minutes and 2 hours to feel 10 movements.
- Count at roughly the same time every day.
- Pick a time of the day when your baby is normally active.
- If for some reason you're not feeling movements as you normally would, have a snack, and then try to count again.
- If movements still aren't normal after eating something, or if it's taking you much longer than before to reach 10, call your healthcare provider or go to the hospital straight away.

night, while others prefer to keep all their active movements for during the day. Most babies move after a meal as the rush of blood sugar hits their system, giving them a boost of energy, while some move before a meal to indicate that they're hungry.

Regardless of the type of baby you have, your late second trimester homework is to pay attention to your baby and figure out what her normal movement pattern is. Once you have that established, you should pay attention to any deviations in the pattern, and if you don't feel normal movements, consult your healthcare provider immediately. While most of the time

> I understand how a baby not moving enough is worrisome, but what about a baby who's moving ALL THE TIME??? #tiredout

everything is fine, it's better that you get the baby checked out to put your mind at rest than to fret about there being something wrong. Your midwife or doctor will probably ask you to visit the hospital for a non-stress test (NST) to confirm that the baby is okay.

The non-stress test

This is a painless, non-invasive test that uses an external foetal heart monitor for 20–30 minutes to evaluate your baby's condition. During this time, the resting baseline of your baby's heart rate is recorded, as well as periods of activity and movement. If your baby is asleep during the test, you may be given a snack or some juice to help wake the baby up.

If you have diabetes, high blood pressure, pre-eclampsia or any other medical condition which affects your pregnancy, your provider may order weekly or bi-weekly NSTs for you, starting as early as 28 weeks. This test is also done if there are any concerns about foetal growth, particularly if your baby has been on the small side, or if there are concerns about the placenta or the quantity of amniotic fluid. If the baby needs to be turned from breech position (rump first) to vertex position (head first) through a process known as an external cephalic version, an NST will be carried out before and after the version. An NST is also usually done in conjunction with a biophysical profile (see below).

Biophysical profile

A biophysical profile (BPP) is a specialized ultrasound scan that measures five distinct attributes in your baby and gives the baby a score for each one. The five attributes examined are the baby's breathing, muscle tone, heart rate, amniotic fluid volume and movement. For example, to assess your baby's 'breathing', the sonographer looks for at least one breathing episode (where your baby's ribcage can be seen expanding and contracting with practice breaths) within a period of 30 minutes. To assess muscle tone, the sonographer looks for one or more episodes of active limb extension, or opening and closing of a hand. For movement, the sonographer looks for two or more movements in 30 minutes (these can be small, fine movements, such as wiggling fingers or torso, tucking the head or stretching the feet). The heart rate is assessed through an NST, and the amniotic fluid is measured to check that it's adequate. Your baby scores 2 for each of the attributes that are looking normal, or zero if the criteria aren't met. On average, a normal BPP score is 10 out of 10, or 8 out of 10 if the NST is not performed.

BPPs can be performed as early as 32 weeks if there is any question about foetal wellbeing, particularly if your baby is on the small side or if there are concerns about the baby's overall health. Although many more women have them towards the end of the pregnancy to assess 'late' babies, or to help decide whether an induction is needed.

Condensed idea
Most tests are to confirm the baby's wellbeing, not to find a problem

29 Breathless and impatient

The final weeks of the pregnancy can be some of the most uncomfortable as the baby continues to grow. But at last the light at the end of the tunnel is visible – your breathlessness, aching back and puffy ankles are really a sign that your due date is fast approaching.

Ways to breathe better

In your third trimester everything gets a little bit harder to do, including catching your breath. It's not because you're in terrible shape – it's because the baby is taking up all of the room your lungs would otherwise use to expand. As the uterus grows, it actually extends up into your ribcage and displaces the diaphragm by almost 5 cm (2 in). Knowing the cause of your breathlessness might make you feel a bit better, and taking slower, deeper breaths might help you too. Concentrating on good posture helps give your lungs a bit more breathing room (this is where exercises like yoga really come in handy), and you can also stretch your arms up over your head or place your hands on your head, both of which will open up your ribcage slightly.

> Feels like I'm sitting in a lake, day and night – please tell me this is normal?!? #preggershelp

If breathlessness bothers you at night when you're trying to sleep, try propping a few pillows under your head and back so you're more upright. For many women this usually gets better in the last few weeks of pregnancy as the baby drops into the pelvis, giving your lungs more breathing room.

Easing backache

Not surprisingly, backache is incredibly common. As the weight of your baby and protruding belly begins to shift your centre of gravity forwards, more pressure is put on your lower back to support your upright position and counterbalance the weight in front. The stretching of the uterus also puts pressure on the ligaments attached to your sacrum (tailbone). Many women also experience upper back pain due to an increase in breast size.

While there's not much you can do to prevent all this, using proper body mechanics may help relieve it somewhat: always bend at the knees, not the back, and keep your feet shoulder-width apart when lifting. Try to avoid excessive bending and lifting (if possible), but if you do need to stand for a long period of time,

> Jimmy Choos? I can't even get my loafers on any more. #barefootmum

rest one foot on a stool, if you can, to relieve back pressure. Make sure you do plenty of stretching exercises throughout the day (lift your arms high over your head every hour or so), wear comfortable, supportive shoes (flats are much better than heels at this stage), and when you're getting up from lying flat on your back, roll to your side and push yourself up with your arms. Getting on all fours and rocking back and forth, or having someone massage or press on your sacrum may also help. Some women find that sleeping on a futon or firmer mattress really makes a difference. If none of this works, switch to comfort measures: warm compresses, nice relaxing baths, a pregnancy abdominal support or brace, massage, acupuncture, chiropractic care and even physiotherapy.

Swollen ankles

When you're pregnant, you hold on to extra fluid, and by the third trimester all of this extra liquid tends to pool in your feet and ankles by the end of the day. This is known as dependent oedema, and while it's

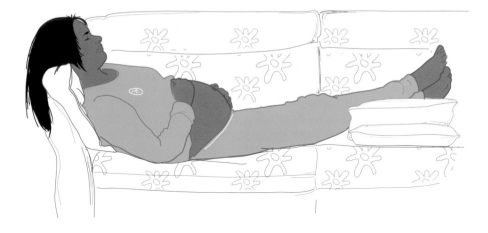

quite common, it's never pleasant (especially in the winter, when the only shoes that fit are your flip-flops). Dependent oedema is also made worse by standing for long periods of time. During the day, try propping your feet up on a foot stool or chair, or lying down on the couch and putting your feet up on the arm (ignore all complaints from others around you!).

At night, take some of your extra pillows and prop your feet up so that they're higher than the level of your heart while you're sleeping. When you wake up in the morning your feet and ankles are usually back to their normal selves. You can also put on a pair of pregnancy support tights first thing in the morning to help maintain this throughout the day.

You may also notice swelling in your hands and fingers – many pregnant women take off their rings towards the end of the pregnancy. Soaking swollen hands and feet in cold water (sometimes with some Epsom salts thrown in) will help relieve the tingling and burning feeling from the stretching skin. Continue to drink plenty of fluids and do not limit your salt intake, as this won't help. However, if excessive swelling comes on very suddenly, or if you have excessive swelling in the face as well, speak with your doctor, as this is sometimes a sign of pre-eclampsia.

What's happened to my skin?

In addition to everything else going on, pregnancy causes a lot of skin changes (which usually disappear after the pregnancy), including:

- The linea nigra – a thin, dark line that runs down the centre of your belly.
- Chloasma – this is a patch of darker pigmentation that often appears on the nose, cheeks and forehead, and is usually worsened by sun exposure.
- Acne – who knew that being pregnant could make you look like a teenager again?
- Spider veins and spider angiomas – red areas where blood vessels show near the surface of the skin.
- PUPPPs (pruritic urticarial papules and plaques of pregnancy) – raised hives and bumps usually on your belly, but sometimes also on your hips, thighs, upper arms and buttocks. These are harmless but incredibly itchy.
- Varicose veins – these may not completely disappear after the pregnancy, but usually get much better (leg elevation and compression stockings will help with this as well).

condensed idea
A big, healthy baby might cause mum some short-lived discomfort

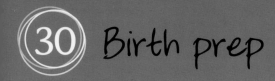

30 Birth prep

While Mother Nature has already endowed you with everything you need to give birth, most people attend a childbirth education class at this stage of the pregnancy. However, birth preparation includes a lot more than formal classes, especially if you're planning a home birth.

The Lamaze method

The Lamaze method single-handedly launched the formal childbirth education movement. Introduced in France in 1951 by the French doctor Fernand Lamaze, its central idea was that if women are taught and frequently practise a series of specific breathing techniques before the birth, these will become automatic responses to contractions. While these breathing techniques are still taught, Lamaze classes now include a much wider philosophy of birth. Unlike some methods, the Lamaze philosophy is open to the taking of pain-relieving drugs, and many women use Lamaze techniques up to the point that they get an epidural.

Husbands and hypnobirthing

Various other methods and techniques arose to help shape modern ideas about birth preparation. For example, the Bradley method, founded by American obstetrician Dr Robert A Bradley in 1965, revolutionized birth practices by teaching 'husband-coached childbirth'. It places a strong emphasis on having the partner present at the birth and playing a crucial supporting role (prior to this, husbands seldom attended the birth).

The Leboyer method, developed in the 1970s by Dr Frederick Leboyer, emphasizes a calm and soothing environment for the baby immediately after the delivery. His ideas about gently welcoming the baby into the world without trauma have changed the way we view the immediate needs of the newborn.

The work of British doctor Grantly Dick-Read during the 1930s cited 'the vicious circle of the fear–tension–pain syndrome' as being responsible for much of the pain of labour. Marie Mongan's hypnobirthing method (see box on page 98) expands on his ideas, teaching deep abdominal breathing, relaxation and self-hypnosis techniques to induce a trance-like state during labour. Those who are able to successfully use the techniques sometimes report completely painless labours.

Another popular childbirth education method, *Birthing From Within*, was developed by midwife Pam England after she had an unwanted caesarean with her first child (the outcome she had most feared prior to

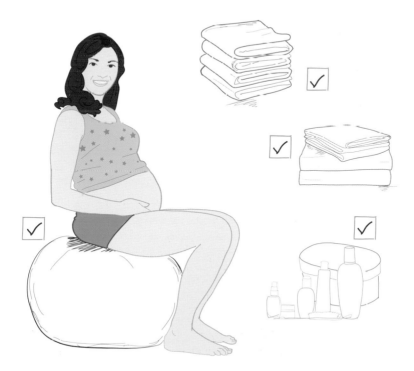

delivering). Hers is a very flexible approach that emphasizes the spiritual aspects of birth rather than just the physical, and teaches a variety of pain coping techniques. These days, most childbirth education classes draw from a variety of sources and tend to give a broad overview without focusing on one specific philosophy or technique.

What to look for in a childbirth class

Childbirth education is a lot more than just learning about how to deal with pain. To help find the right class for you, consider the following:

- Research the course instructor's qualifications, experience and training. Is this someone who knows what she's talking about? It might help to talk to her on the phone as well. Do you like her personal style? Is she interesting and engaging?
- Find out who the instructor works for. Is he an independent teacher, or does he work for the hospital or a health authority? If he works for the hospital and you are planning a home birth, for example, it might not be the best fit.
- Does the class teach a specific method or philosophy? If so, which one? Does the content of this method fit with what you're looking for from your birth experience? (If you're planning on an epidural, for example, you'll want a class which covers medical pain-relief options as well as natural childbirth.)
- Find out the specifics of the class: how large will it be? Is it designed for your birth support team too, or just the pregnant couple? Will labour techniques be practised in class? Does it also cover breastfeeding and newborn care? How many weeks does it last? How much does it cost?

Get the bag packed, ready to go

For hospital births, it's a good idea to pack your bag well in advance of your due date. Put in your bathrobe, slippers, a comfy change of clothes, toiletries and a set of clothes for the baby. If you've been given a copy of your antenatal chart, be sure to bring that as well, plus anything else you think you'd want for the delivery (such as a

> Uh oh. I was the only person in class today raising her hand for major pain relief during labour. #mydeliverychoice

birth ball, music or a hot-water bottle). But keep to labour requirements – you won't need the baby car seat, for instance, until you're ready to go home, so someone else can bring that to the hospital later.

Getting ready for a home birth

Birth preparation also includes prepping your home if you're planning to give birth there. Most home-birth midwives will give you a list of everything you will need for your home birth. This usually involves getting a birth kit from your midwife or online (these kits usually contain gloves, pads, gauze, antiseptic wipes and anything else your midwife will require at the birth, aside from her own surgical tools, oxygen and resuscitation equipment, which she will bring herself). You'll also need plenty of spare sheets and towels which you don't mind getting dirty, and a plastic mattress cover for your bed to go under the sheets. Sometimes a plastic shower curtain or painting dustsheet also works well to help protect your furniture or carpet.

Condensed idea
Being prepared means you'll feel more confident on the big day

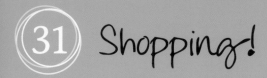

31 Shopping!

The amount of baby stuff out there can be overwhelming, especially for first-time parents. What are your actual baby needs, versus baby wants? While it's fun to go a bit crazy, you'd be surprised to learn that babies need a lot less than some firms would like you to think.

Decisions, decisions

While some eager couples start shopping from the moment they hear the news, other couples feel like it's bad luck to shop for a baby before she's born, and for others it doesn't even dawn on them until well into the third trimester that having a baby requires a whole lot of brand new gear. Before you hit the panic button and run to your local baby store in a frenzy, though, consider this: you can always buy the bare minimum now, and then make other purchases along the way once you get a better idea of what you actually need for your baby. Many items that stores insist are essential, such as a high-chair, won't be needed until your baby is around 6 months old, so you have more time than you may think.

> Mum's gone mad in the baby shop. She's left me nothing to buy baby myself! #thwartedshopper

Cradle or cot?

One thing you will definitely need from the very beginning is somewhere for the baby to sleep. Some couples like to buy a full-size cot that will also convert into a toddler bed, while others will use a bassinet (cradle) or Moses basket for the first few months before switching to the larger cot once the baby's older. The first option saves you money in the long term, since you'll only be buying one item, but tiny babies don't need that much room in the beginning, and many couples quickly discover that they want their newborn much closer to them than the cot will allow.

The essential shopping list

While you can certainly add to this, these are the basics which you should have in place before the arrival of your baby:

- Crib/bassinet/cot/Moses basket – somewhere for the baby to sleep.
- Fitted sheets to cover the mattress (two sets so that you can wash one while the other is in use).
- Nappies and wipes.
- Changing pad (this can be as simple as a mat which you lay out on the floor; the floor is actually a great place to change a baby, as there's no way she can roll off it!)
- Infant bath.
- First aid kit, including bulb syringe, thermometer, safety scissors/nail clippers, alcohol wipes, cotton buds (for cleaning around the umbilical cord, not for the baby's ears).
- Bottles and sterilizing equipment.
- Baby clothes (lots of 'onesies' and babygrows).
- Swaddling blankets (your baby will love being swaddled in the first months).
- A nappy bag (not truly essential, but incredibly handy).
- A car seat.

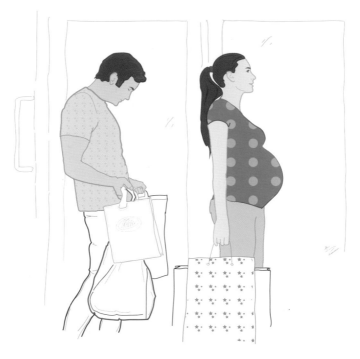

The advantage of the bassinet or Moses basket is that they are both very small, and can be placed in your room right next to your bed, which makes going to your newborn in the middle of the night much easier. Many couples also choose to use a co-sleeper in the beginning, which is a small bassinette that actually attaches to the side of the bed like a motorcycle side-car and allows your baby to be not feet but inches away from you without any danger of you rolling over on top of her.

Regardless of what you decide upon, it's imperative that you don't place any bumpers, pillows or stuffed animals around the crib, as all of these items can increase the likelihood of sudden infant ieath syndrome (SIDS). The NHS in Britain and the American Academy of Paediatrics in the USA do not recommend sharing your bed with your baby as this also increases the chance of SIDS. If you plan on co-sleeping, opt for the side-car attachment instead. Blankets and sheets have also been implicated in instances of SIDS, so buy a baby sleeping bag, which prevents your baby from getting anything tangled around her head at night.

Car seats and buggies

Another item you won't be able to skimp on is the car seat. While there are thousands of different models out there, with prices ranging from less than £100 to over £300, each of them has met the minimum safety standard, and most hospitals require you to leave with your baby in a car seat. If you're looking at pushchairs now, you might consider buying a frame which your car seat can snap into and using it as your starter pushchair – car seat and buggy at the same time! Or you may choose to ignore buggies altogether; there are hundreds of models of soft carriers and wraps available that allow parents to wear their babies instead, and in the first few months, being snuggled close to a parent is incredibly reassuring to a baby.

Nappy dilemmas

While it may seem like there isn't much to decide on in the nappy department, you might be surprised to learn that you'll go through around 3,000 of them a year, so actually it is rather a big decision. While disposable nappies are without a doubt the easiest to use, they are made of synthetic materials and plastic, and will take approximately 500 years to break down in landfill. There are now a few brands of eco-nappies, which are pricier but biodegradeable. Cloth nappies are definitely more time-intensive, but they're reusable and leave no landfill waste, and your baby will probably be potty trained at a younger age, because she will become quickly aware of being wet. There are also many firms now specializing in laundering cloth nappies. Or you can get the best of both worlds, perhaps, with a hybrid nappy – a cloth cover which uses a flushable lining.

Condensed idea
Baby shopping can seem intimidating, so focus on the essentials

(32) Pre-birth celebrations

Pregnancy is a really special time in your life, and you'll probably want to celebrate it in some way. In some countries, the baby shower is a popular tradition, while many other cultures have celebrations and rituals to honour the pregnancy itself.

Baby showers

The modern baby shower developed shortly after World War II during the baby-boom era. It was seen as the perfect opportunity to shower the new family with baby-related gifts, thereby lessening the economic burden placed on the couple, but it also fitted hand-in-hand with the consumerism of the 1950s. Traditionally, a baby shower is a women-only event. Refreshments are served, the expectant woman is placed on a central (often decorated) chair, and the piles of presents are opened by her one by one, with each item admired and passed around by the guests. A playful atmosphere, music and games (like guessing the gender or name of the baby) are also usually part of this custom. These days, many baby showers are given for the couple rather than just the woman, so men also attend the party; the chair and games may or may not be present, and alcoholic beverages are served rather than just fruit punch and soft drinks. Some baby showers even involve DJs and dancing, and can be large and lavish affairs.

In the USA, the tradition of baby showers has grown alongside the tradition of registering for baby gifts – in the same way that you might register a list of gifts for your wedding. A baby gift registry ensures that all of the baby gifts you receive are actually items you would like to own, making it very easy for family and friends to buy gifts for you – most of

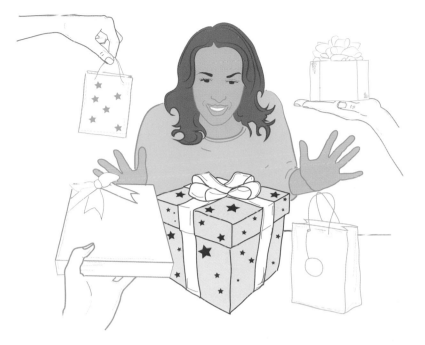

whom can't wait to get shopping! There's no duplication of gifts, and non-parents are relieved to know they're giving something genuinely useful. Registries can be set up online or in stores.

Blessingway ceremonies

In the last decade or so, a more feminist spin on the baby shower has emerged, known as a Blessingway (or Mother Blessing). While baby showers tend to be focused on the baby, and in particular on material items the couple will need once the baby is born, the Blessingway is all about nurturing the mother-to-be and honouring the rite of passage she's about to undergo. The idea of a Blessingway is based loosely on an American-Indian Navajo tradition and has no set custom – you are free to create whatever kind of ritual is meaningful to you. Usually it's a women-only event, with the mum-to-be surrounded by her most trusted friends and female loved ones.

The Mother Blessing

The purpose of this gathering is to recognize your rite of passage, from woman to mother, and to support you during the transition. You're free to use any, all or none of the ideas – what's important is that you feel a growing sense of support.

- Ask each of the guests to bring a small bead with them, and a prayer or wish for you during labour. Then string all of the beads together to make a bracelet or necklace, and wear it during the birth as a physical reminder of all of the support you have.
- Sit in a circle and pass a ball of red thread to each other across the circle as each woman shares her own birth experience or wishes for your childbirth, creating a visual web of connection. Ask each woman to tie a piece of the thread around her wrist and wear it until you give birth.
- Ask the women to decorate your belly with henna or paint, or make a belly cast – messy, but incredible fun, and a wonderful keepsake for you to remember your beautiful pregnant body. (Henna skin-painting is a tradition within many cultures and has been used on pregnant women for centuries.)
- Mother the mother – guests can massage you, brush your hair, give you a foot bath and rub, paint your toenails and so on while you curl up in the loving embrace of your circle.
- At the end of the ceremony, give every participant a tall votive candle, and ask them to light it when they hear that you're in labour, and keep it burning until you give birth. While you're in labour, you can imagine the lit flames of your loved ones keeping vigil for you.

There may be a central poem or reading; each woman may share stories from her own birth and experiences she's had with children or as a parent; or she may offer up hopes, wishes and blessings for the upcoming birth. A Blessingway honours all belief systems and often provides a safe space for the expectant woman to ground herself, release any concerns or fears she has about the birth, and

> Feeling totally empowered after Mother Blessing and feel like maybe I can actually do this. Big thanks to all. #newmama

celebrate and embrace her future role as a mother. There are countless ways to celebrate a Blessingway, but we've put together some starter ideas for you in the box opposite.

New (pregnant) friends

Like all rites of passage, it's impossible to fully understand the complexities of becoming a mum until you've been through it yourself, which is why meeting other pregnant and new-mum friends is so crucial. In the new and wondrous (and sleepless) months which lie ahead of you, few will be able to empathize the way another brand-new mother can. New-mum friends will give you a sympathetic ear, another perspective, and an instant circle of support Which means that next time you see another pregnant woman at your local café or supermarket, say hi! Ask her when her due date is, find out if she lives nearby, and keep in touch; when you both have young babies, it will be an instant play date! Childbirth education classes and antenatal exercise classes are also great places to make new friends.

Condensed idea
Celebrating your pregnancy is an important part of becoming a mother

(33) The waiting game

Only five per cent of women give birth on their actual due date – many more go overdue. Those last few weeks of pregnancy can seem interminable; everything is ready, the only thing missing is the baby! Nevertheless, try to enjoy your last few weeks – there's no need to rush.

Make the most of it

You've made it! You're now officially full term, and your baby's due to arrive at any moment, but the question is… when will that moment be? In most normal, healthy pregnancies, you're looking at a five-week window of readiness, from 37 weeks to 42 weeks (remember, 40 weeks is the due date), during which time you can spontaneously go into labour at any point.

It's hard to remain patient at this point, but just keep reminding yourself that the whole process of labour will work better if your body has activated it spontaneously. There are of course some natural things you can do to try to give your body a nudge (see the box opposite for some suggestions), but the last few weeks of pregnancy are all about acceptance – recognizing that your baby has his own timetable, and that you're exactly where you need to be: waiting. The days of your pregnancy are numbered, so try to make the most of them. It will never again be so easy to take your baby with you everywhere you go; in only a few short weeks (or days) you'll no longer get to feel him moving and wiggling within your body, carried beneath your heart. Soon enough that large and lovely belly of yours will be gone, not to mention your free time, so try to enjoy all of this while you've still got it, because your life will never be the same again!

Now is the time to go out for long and luxurious dinners with your partner. Catch up on all those movies you've been wanting to see, because seeing a movie together (and uninterrupted) will become a much rarer thing once the baby arrives. If you were considering making a belly cast, or having a pregnancy photography session done, now is the time. Go out in the evenings, enjoy each other's company, make love,

Get the ball rolling!

While patience is a virtue, it's natural to want to do something to try to bring on labour. The list below offers some time-honoured tricks, but speak with your doctor or midwife before trying any of them, because every pregnancy is different.

- Sex, sex and more sex. Semen is a great source of prostaglandins, which help soften and ripen the cervix.
- Acupuncture can work wonders for getting labour going.
- Begin taking evening primrose oil, a source of omega-6 fatty acids that are converted into several beneficial substances in the body, including prostaglandin. You can take two 500 mg capsules orally 2–3 times a day.
- If you're over 39 weeks, mix 50 g (2 oz) of castor oil with 2 cups of orange juice and 2 scoops of vanilla ice cream, blend and drink, and then follow up with hot peppermint tea. Castor oil irritates the intestines, which in turn irritates the uterus and begins contractions. However, be prepared to spend some quality time in the bathroom after you've taken the castor oil, as it frequently causes diarrhoea (and definitely talk about trying this with your healthcare provider before giving it a go).

and sleep now as much as you can. In fact, studies have shown that the better rested you are before your labour, the shorter your labour will be (on average), so don't feel even remotely guilty about turning over and going back to sleep for an extra few hours every morning. Once the baby arrives, this is one luxury that you won't be able to revel in for a while.

Counting movements

If you go past your due date, it's important that you perform your foetal movement counting daily (see page 113), and be extra-attentive during this time. Tell your midwife or doctor immediately if you notice any decrease in movement, so that they can carry out thorough checks (such as the BPP profile; see page 115). The concern here is that the placenta can start to get tired once it's older than 40 weeks, which may result in decreased amniotic fluid. In this scenario, your doctor or midwife is likely to offer you an induction to begin labour, rather than wait for spontaneous labour to begin.

However, in the majority of cases, tests are used to reassure your healthcare team (as well as you) that everything is looking good and it's okay to continue to wait for spontaneous labour to begin. While an induction might sound like an easier and faster option (it will put an end to the waiting, after all), in reality it is likely to be a very long and difficult process. Inductions can sometimes last as long as 2–3 days.

> This pregnancy is like a lesson in patience. Come on baby, let's get going! #readymum

Studies have shown that women who are induced have increased rates of medical intervention in addition to an increased chance of needing a caesarean birth as well. In general, as long as everything is looking good with your baby and your doctor or midwife is happy with the way things are going, waiting for your body to go into labour on its own is always the best bet.

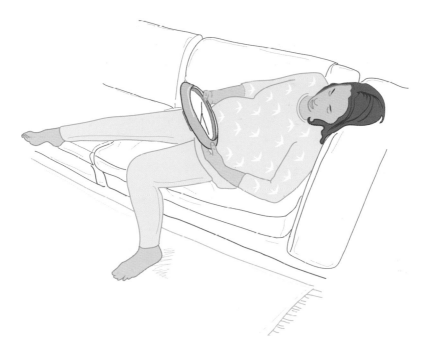

Nesting

If you're finding it hard to enjoy your last few weeks, try to distract yourself instead: break out the board games, catch up on a TV series, finish your novel, get a pedicure, play cards or work on a craft project. But beware of sudden, intense urges to clean and organize everything in sight! This phenomenon, known as 'the nesting instinct', is a sudden burst of energy which usually comes a day or two before you go into labour (and sometimes just a few hours before labour). Many women find themselves strangely drawn to mopping every floor in their house, cleaning out the attic or re-organizing their cupboards. If you find yourself feeling this way, try your best to ignore it and rest instead.

Condensed idea
**While waiting is never easy,
labour has its own schedule**

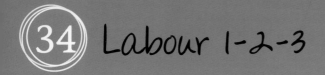

34 Labour 1-2-3

No two labours are the same, but there are four distinct phases of labour that every woman goes through. There's really no way of explaining quite how labour feels, but this chapter will serve as a broad overview for each stage and its variations.

First stage

The first stage of labour is what most people think of when they think of labour. It involves effacement (thinning) and dilation (opening) of the cervix, and covers the start of contractions up until the point when you're fully dilated and ready to push, which marks the beginning of the second stage. Even though the first stage is divided into two phases (latent phase and active phase), these are arbitrary designations used to help your doctor and midwife assess your progress, and in reality the first stage is a continuous process, with one phase blending into the next.

During the latent phase, also known as early labour, the cervix begins to dilate and efface, moving from zero to 3–4 cm dilation, and contractions are generally mild, irregular and spaced far apart (coming every 10–15 minutes). The latent phase can last anywhere from a few hours to days, and it's even possible for contractions to start and stop during this time. Early labour can be particularly difficult, as the contractions are often uncomfortable and usually frequent enough to prevent sleep, but most hospitals won't admit you until you hit the active phase (which starts from 3–4 cm onwards), so you still have to find a way to cope until then.

Once the active phase begins, the contractions usually become a lot closer together (every 2–4 minutes), last longer and are much stronger and more intense. At this point the cervix begins to dilate far more rapidly, and labour now requires all of your concentration. During the active phase, the presenting part of the foetus (usually the baby's head) begins to descend lower into the pelvis. If your bag of waters hasn't broken yet, it usually does so during the active phase. The very end of the active phase, right before you begin pushing, is known as transition. This usually starts at around 8–9 cm dilation, and is characterized by extremely intense and frequent contractions. Many women may also vomit, hiccup, burp and shake, and can become irritable, restless and despairing, but in fact these signs are very encouraging, indicating that you've just about finished with the first stage and are about to begin the second.

The length of the first stage of labour can vary tremendously. It can last for days, or be as short as just a few (very intense) hours. For first-time mums, the average length of the active phase of labour is 8 hours, although even a 16-hour active phase is still considered normal. For women who've already had a baby before, the active phase is much shorter, lasting 5 hours on average.

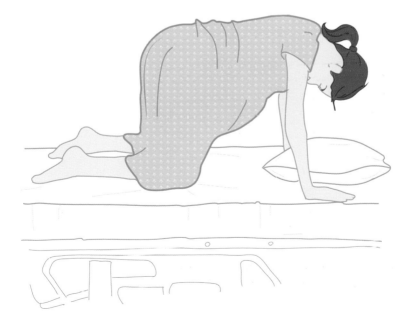

What will labour feel like?

When you've never experienced labour before and the closest
you've been to it is watching screaming women acting out
childbirth on TV, it's really hard to know what to expect. Some
women describe contractions as rushes of energy (including
the famous midwifery pioneer Ina May Gaskin); other women
describe them as squeezing, grinding or twisting. If you've had
bad menstrual cramps before, you may try to imagine them as
really, really strong cramps. But before you make up your mind
about labour before you've experienced it, consider this:

• You can think of each contraction as a wave,
  starting slowly, gradually building to a crescendo,
  and then fading again.
• Each pain consists of the uterus flexing and then
  resting. During the peak of a contraction, you
  can feel the muscle of your uterus ball up like a
  rock, become hard, then gradually relax again (it's
  similar to the way your bicep balls up and becomes
  rock hard when flexed, then relaxes again). Each
  flex of the uterus works to pull the cervix open,
  little by little.
• In the beginning, contractions last 20–30 seconds,
  and gradually increase in duration and frequency
  until they're lasting for a minute, and coming every
  2–3 minutes during transition.
• The pain of labour is really well designed. Yes, it's
  very intense, but not constant. There are built-in
  rest breaks between every contraction – a chance
  to catch your breath before the next surge.

Second stage

The second stage of labour begins once you're fully dilated and ready to push, and lasts up until the birth of the baby. During this stage, the contractions change slightly, becoming stronger at the top of the uterus in an effort to push the baby down and out. Most women who don't have an epidural usually feel an overwhelming urge to push along with their contractions during this time, and the combined force is able to expel the baby. The second stage can be as fast as one or two pushes (especially if this is not your first baby), or as long as two to three hours. If your waters haven't broken, or been broken by your midwife, they normally break on their own while you're pushing.

> I laboured for 16 hours and boy was it painful but I forgot it all when I saw her face.
> #alldoneanddusted

Third and fourth stage

The third stage lasts from the time of the delivery of the baby up until the delivery of the placenta (afterbirth), which slowly separates from the uterine wall and is gently eased out by your midwife or doctor. The contractions slow down and are much milder than they were before. This stage can be as short as just a few minutes, or as long as 45 minutes to an hour. The fourth stage – the first hour after delivery of the placenta – is known as the recovery stage, when your body is rapidly adjusting to its now not-pregnant state. In most healthy women, recovery goes smoothly, but your midwife or doctor will still be monitoring you closely during this time.

Condensed idea
Each woman goes through four distinct phases during labour and birth

You're often so caught up in labour that you're not even aware of the passage of time. Your body is built for labour, though, so however long it feels, remember that most labours progress perfectly on their own given enough time and patience.

What kick-starts labour?

We still don't fully understand what actually causes labour to begin. One idea is that the foetus itself sends a signal to the mother's body that triggers the release of oxytocin and prostaglandins, two of the hormones responsible for orchestrating contractions. Another theory suggests that

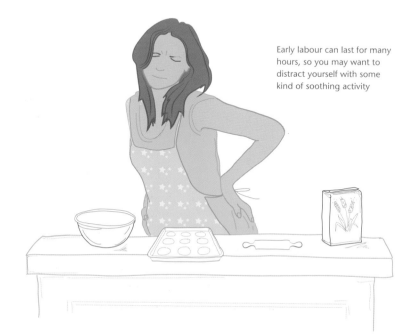

Early labour can last for many hours, so you may want to distract yourself with some kind of soothing activity

there are stretch receptors built into the muscle of the uterus which trigger the start of labour when the baby reaches a certain size, but obviously this varies greatly. We do know that more labours begin at night than during the day, perhaps because the body can finally relax enough to allow labour to start once the bustles and demands of the day are over.

Early labour

Some labours start in a relaxed and leisurely manner, while others begin like a horse out of a gate. For most first-time mums, though, early labour can be a very long process. During early labour your cervix is softening and slowly beginning to dilate (see page 136), but contractions are often still irregular. Naturally you're excited by these early contractions, and may start to time them immediately and get ready for the birth. But in most cases there's no need to rush to the hospital. If you have a history of very rapid labours, you might

> Midwife says these false contractions are helping me to get ready for the real deal. I'm ready already! #letsgetgoing

want to call your midwife or doctor a bit sooner, but if this is your first time, usually there's no need to check in until the contractions are uncomfortable and coming every 5 minutes or so. Until then, it's better to try to relax, distract yourself as much as you can and wait to see what happens. If you're really in labour, it will become obvious soon enough.

It might help to make a list of activities you can do during early labour to help take your mind off it, such as baking, knitting or watching TV. Choose an activity that gives you time to pause and breathe through a contraction every now and then. Early labour is also a great time to practise your relaxation techniques: slow, deep breathing; having a massage, shower or bath; listening to music; meditating or practising visualization. It's also important to keep yourself hydrated during this time, so make sure you have a selection of drinks in the house to sip

What to do when your waters break

Most women's waters will break during labour. This is usually an obvious event, but in some women it can appear as a slow trickle rather than a pouring tap.

- Call your midwife or doctor to let them know.
- Most of the time the fluid is clear, with a slight alkaline smell, but occasionally it can be brownish or greenish in colour if it's meconium-stained (this happens when the baby empties her bowels into the amniotic fluid – usually a sign of foetal stress).
- If you're unsure whether your waters have broken or not, put on a pad and check it after an hour; if you have indeed broken your waters, the pad is usually soaked. A pad might be useful anyway to keep yourself dry.
- Once your waters break, be sure to avoid sex and/or putting anything inside your vagina.
- In 8–12 per cent of all births, the waters break before labour has even started, a condition known as premature rupture of membranes (PROM). Your doctor or midwife will want to see you or perhaps send you to hospital to confirm the rupture. If left alone, most women will spontaneously go into labour within 24 hours of PROM, but induction may be recommended sooner than that.

on. The same goes for food; have small snacks of complex carbs and proteins, not sugars. If contractions begin in the middle of the night, try to sleep between them, or at least stay in bed, resting. Anything you can do now to conserve your energy will be helpful once active labour starts.

You may also lose your 'mucus plug' at this time. This brown and stretchy 'plug' is the dense matrix of mucus in the cervix that has protected the baby from ascending bacteria during the pregnancy (some women even lose their plug a day or two before labour begins), and is always considered a very encouraging sign. You may also notice pink-tinged vaginal secretions, known as 'show'. As the cervix stretches and begins to dilate, it often bleeds slightly, causing the pink discharge; this is a good sign as it means your contractions are having an effect on your cervix.

Time to move

Most women are able to chat in between contractions during early labour, but as the contractions become stronger and you shift into active labour, your concentration becomes focused inwards, and even simple things like speaking or following a conversation become difficult. It's time to call your doctor or midwife, or head to the hospital, when your contractions are regular (every 5 minutes) and strong, if your waters break or if you notice any heavy, bright-red vaginal bleeding.

False labour

Sometimes you may go through false labour before the real deal. False labour consists of contractions that don't actually cause cervical dilation; they remain irregular and short, but can be every bit as exhausting. True contractions will gradually become more regular, frequent and intense over time. To tell them apart, go for a walk. Usually walking will ease the contractions of false labour, or even make them go away, while with true labour walking tends to make the contractions more intense. Monitor the signs and be sure to keep your midwife up to date.

Condensed idea
Early labour can be a long process, so try to relax and rest for as long as you can

36 Keeping it natural

Labour is a very personal journey and there is no right or wrong way to get through it, but some women remain deeply committed to having a natural childbirth. If this appeals to you, there are many effective, natural pain coping techniques at your disposal.

Working with the pain

With natural childbirth, there's no way to avoid the pain – and in fact, there are many researchers and authors who suggest the pain of labour is both healthy and necessary. According to midwife and author Pam England, the pain of labour helps release stress hormones, which help prevent hypoxia (insufficient oxygen) in your baby as well as preparing his lungs to breathe. Pain also helps guide a woman in labour; the positions she naturally chooses to help cope with the pain are often the perfect positions to promote labour progress and help the baby descend into the pelvis. When you remove the pain of labour – as with an epidural – you often remove these positive feedback loops, so labour often lasts longer and requires augmentation with synthetic oxytocin (see pages 150–51).

Mental preparation, a lack of fear, a positive attitude and great support all play a crucial role in coping successfully with pain. Author Penny Simkin has written extensively about the difference between pain and suffering. A long, painful labour is not necessarily a cause for suffering; it's hard work, certainly, but pain is not always a bad thing. Childbirth educator Beth Donnelly Caban suggests we reframe our ideas about labour pain through 'the five Ps'. Labour is painful, but it's a Positive sign. Increasing pain and intensity is usually an indication of Progress.

Labour pain is also Purposeful – it's accomplishing something, rather than being a sign of disease. Contractions are also Periodic, so you can get your breath back, and Predictable, giving you time to prepare and creating a useful rhythm.

Activate the right nervous system

Pain, and often the fear of pain, causes a great deal of tension in the body. The more you tense in response to the contractions, the more painful they become. The more you can relax, and keep all of the rest of your muscles in a relaxed state, the easier the contractions are to bear. Breath serves as the crux of relaxation. Slow, deep breaths automatically activate your parasympathetic nervous system (responsible for rest

Back labour

Back labour occurs when the baby is facing up instead of down, which puts the hard bony parts of the baby's head against the hard bony parts of your sacrum and spine. The result is often excruciating, and back labours are often longer and slower, as the baby has to rotate into a more optimal position in order to be born. If you're in back labour, try moving on to your hands and knees, as this position encourages the baby to rotate, and takes some of the pressure off your back. Or you could ask someone to perform either:

• Counterpressure – strong, constant pressure against your sacrum or lower back during a contraction, usually with the heel of the hand.
• The double hip squeeze – firm, constant pressure applied to either side of your hips.

and renewal) instead of your sympathetic nervous system (responsible for fight or flight). It also ensures that you and your baby stay well oxygenated during the labour. Ask your support team to watch for signs of tensed muscles, and to talk you through actively relaxing them between contractions. It also helps to blow air out between your lips like a horse, and to try to keep your mouth and jaw relaxed. As midwife Ina May Gaskin famously says, 'loose lips, loose perineum'.

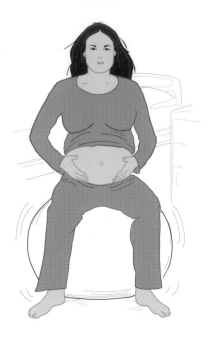

Talking and moving

Making noise during labour can be incredibly helpful, so long as it's a low-pitched noise in your chest and belly (high-pitched noises in the throat and mouth can elicit a kind of panic response in your body). Deep moaning, groaning, chanting or humming are all useful noises, and can be timed with the exhalation of your breath for maximum relaxation, almost as if you're expelling all of the tension from your body with breath and sound combined. Visualization during this time is also incredibly helpful (it works much better if you've practised it before the labour). This involves constructing a mental image in your mind, such as your cervix thinning and opening, or your body relaxing and letting go. The mind is a powerful thing and mind over matter can work wonders where pain is concerned.

Combining your breath with movement is also a fantastic way to get through a contraction. Many women naturally find themselves falling into a rhythm of breathing and moaning while swaying, tapping, rocking or counting. Try bouncing or swaying on a birthing ball, rocking on hands and knees, walking, leaning on a partner or the back of a chair, even squatting – they all work wonders. Any rhythmic pattern will help you cope, but listen to your body to avoid getting stuck in a pattern when it's time to change position.

Water therapy

The use of water in labour is one of the best natural analgesics available, and research has shown it doesn't increase the risk of intrauterine infection. Soaking in a tub often allows you to fully relax in between contractions, with the warmth and weightlessness easing away tension and pain. Keep the water at a sensible temperature – if the tub is too hot (higher than 37°C/99°F), it can

> I leaned on Jack for about 4 hours apparently. Poor bloke could barely stand to hold baby! #busymum

raise the core temperature of both you and the baby. If you don't have access to a bath, pull a chair into the shower and sit with the hot water directed at your back or belly while you lean over the back of the chair.

And remember...

This is just the tip of the iceberg. Check websites for information on other effective, natural pain relief techniques, such as massage, aromatherapy, acupuncture and acupressure, transcutaneous electrical nerve stimulation (TENS) units, the use of hot and cold packs, hypnosis, and stroking and touching the skin lightly (effleurage). The important thing is to practise your pain coping techniques well before labour actually starts.

Condensed idea
Remember that the pain has a purpose and try to work with it

Asking for help

Pain relief during labour has come a long way and these days most epidurals can relieve nearly all of the sensations of labour (which can be a mixed blessing, especially during pushing). But like any medication, there are always risks and side effects to consider.

Why not?

Labour is hard, painful work, but you should never be forced to suffer or endure more than you are able to cope with. The decision to use pain-relief medication in labour is an incredibly personal one, and should be made without pressure, guilt or regret. After all, no one else can know exactly what it is you're feeling – this is your decision to make, and yours alone.

However, it's usually impossible to avoid feeling any pain at all, as early labour can be quite painful, so it's a good idea to practise a few natural pain coping techniques in any case. Also, pushing is sometimes perceived as painful even with an epidural on board. Be open to the journey of birth, and be prepared to change plan as needed. You might have been planning on an epidural, for instance, only to discover that you're too dilated by the time you get to the hospital, and there isn't time. Conversely, you might have been dead-set on natural childbirth, but after two days of labour, an epidural might be just what you need to finally relax and dilate.

> Five minutes ago, agony. Now, absolute bliss. I think I may have fallen in love with my anaesthetist. #blissedout

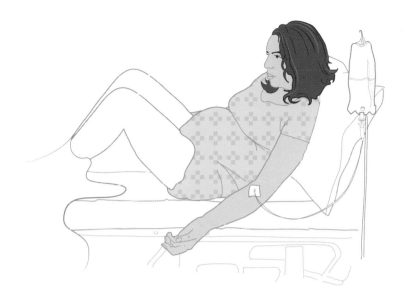

Pain relief through a drip

Most painkillers that are delivered intravenously (directly into a vein) are narcotics derived from the opium poppy, such as morphine and pethidine. In many cases, they are administered with other drugs to prevent nausea and vomiting, as opium-derived drugs often cause nausea as a side-effect. Intravenous painkillers help take the edge off pain, which should help you relax and cope more easily with the contractions. They also tend to cause drowsiness, rather than the euphoria and 'high' feeling that is sometimes associated with narcotics.

The idea behind their use here is to relieve the pain enough to give you a break, without completely knocking you out or wiping your memory away. However, everyone responds differently to these drugs, and you may find yourself feeling 'out of it' for the short time that the drug is at its peak. Most women find themselves sleeping between contractions, perhaps waking up slightly at the very height of the contraction, then drifting off again as the contraction subsides. Side effects of these drugs can include nausea, itching, lowered blood pressure, headache, and, very rarely, respiratory depression; narcotics also cross the placenta, so the baby will be feeling the effects as well. Unlike an epidural, these drugs are relatively short-acting, usually lasting only for 2–3 hours. If given too early, the drugs can sometimes slow down contractions, and their effects on the baby need to wear off before the birth, since they can potentially cause respiratory problems. Your healthcare provider will be well aware of all this, so there's no need to worry.

Gas and air

This is a very popular method of pain relief used in many countries around the world, with the exception of the USA. The colourless, odourless gas nitrous oxide (also known as 'laughing gas') is inhaled combined with oxygen via a mask. You are given the mask and can decide how much or how little to breathe in at any time. Like narcotics, nitrous oxide lessens rather than eliminates pain, but unlike narcotics, it doesn't cross the placenta and it is incredibly short-acting. It can be used at any point in your labour – even while pushing. However, it's not an incredibly strong pain reliever and can occasionally cause drowsiness, nausea and vomiting, a painful tingly feeling or muscle cramps.

Regional anaesthesia

Regional anaesthesia is usually the most effective form of pain relief available during labour, sometimes able to remove all discomfort for hours at a time. The most commonly used form is the epidural, where a constant flow of medication is delivered via a small catheter placed between two vertebrae in your lower back. Once the epidural is in place, you generally become numb from the breasts down; this often limits your ability to walk, and depending on hospital protocol you may be required to stay in bed after the epidural. There are many variations on this, such as the walking epidural, which tends to be a lower dose.

This form of anaesthesia has become incredibly routine these days, but bear in mind that side effects and potential risks always exist whenever an invasive procedure is performed. Common side effects

Do epidurals hinder labour?

The complete pain relief that an epidural provides makes it an attractive option during labour, but it is worth noting the following:

- Women with epidurals often require synthetic oxytocin to help with their contractions.
- An epidural makes pushing more difficult, because you're unable to feel when to push. In some cases, the epidural must be stopped in order to allow the woman to regain enough sensation to push effectively.
- Epidurals have been linked to an increased likelihood of vacuum and forceps use.
- Epidurals are thought to increase the probability of having a caesarean delivery.

include shaking, itching and fever. Epidurals have been known to lower maternal blood pressure, which can affect blood transfer to the baby, and occasionally they cause decelerations in the foetal heart rate. Rarely (in less than one per cent), epidurals can lead to severe headaches and infection is always a risk. Very occasionally, epidurals don't work adequately to numb all pain, and you may require additional pain relief or a repeat epidural. As with all your pregnancy decisions, your choice of pain relief requires careful, informed consideration.

condensed idea
Don't suffer in silence – there are lots of ways to ease the pain

38 The big push

Whether the first stage of your labour was a long, slow marathon or a two-hour runaway train, once you're fully dilated – it's time to push! The second stage of labour brings its own challenges, but at least it helps to know that the birth of your baby is imminent.

A baby on the move

The second stage of labour lasts from being fully dilated right through to delivery. During this stage, the baby's head descends deeper into the pelvis, often rotating to find the perfect path, sometimes 'moulding' as well – this is when the bones of the baby's head shift slightly and sometimes even overlap to allow the head to fit. The soft tissue along the sutures of the baby's skull are designed for this very purpose.

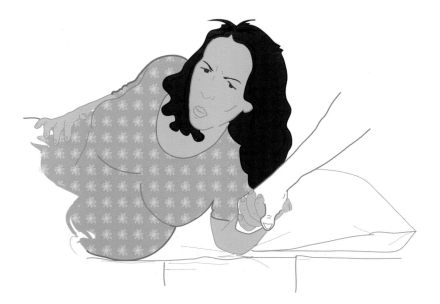

During the birth, the baby travels through eight distinct steps as she moves down towards the birth canal and into the world. These are known as the 'mechanisms of labour' and several of them can occur at once, such as when the baby's head both descends and flexes: the baby moves down through the pelvis while tucking her chin against her chest to present the smallest part of her skull first. Once the baby's head has engaged in the pelvis, it will internally rotate and then 'crown', which refers to the point when the head is visible in the opening of the vagina. Birth occurs by extension of the baby's head, followed by external rotation, which allows the shoulders to rotate and emerge. Usually once the head (the largest part of the baby) is delivered, the rest of the body follows very quickly, often slipping out easily without much effort at all.

One minute I thought it would never end, and then it was all over! Hello baby! #intense

With each contraction, the baby moves down a little bit at a time, often slipping backwards slightly between contractions, which is why it can sometimes feel like taking two steps forwards and one step back. However, this gradual descent gives the baby more time to rotate and find the optimal route through the pelvis. The entire process can take anywhere from 30 minutes to 2–3 hours, especially for first-time mums.

Get pushing!

Like labour, pushing will be different for every woman, every time. The nature of the contractions often begins to change after transition, once you're fully dilated, switching the focus from dilation to expulsion. Many women start to feel incredible pressure in their perineum and rectum, which in many cases mimics the feeling many of us have when we suddenly need to have a bowel movement (this is caused by the baby's head descending even deeper into the vagina and putting more pressure against the rectum). If left on their own, most women will begin to hold

Instinctive pushing

Unless you've been specifically coached to use an active pushing method (which often involves holding your breath and pushing for as long and hard as possible during the contraction), you will probably find yourself using the physiologic method instead. This involves listening to your body's cues and pushing when and how your body tells you that you should. This often amounts to pushing in shorter 'grunts' rather than long, sustained pushes. While overall this method may take a bit longer, since there are fewer pushes per contraction, it also allows greater blood flow and oxygen to your baby during the second stage, and also helps prevent tearing.

their breath and push with the contractions, often referred to as 'bearing down'. In a way, we've been practising our pushing technique all our lives. We've all experienced moments when having a bowel movement where we have this urge, and that often sums up what pushing feels like: your body begins to strain and push with or without you, and it's impossible to stop. The combined force of your own pushing efforts on top of the contractions is what eventually gets the baby out (although pushing only during the contraction is very important, to keep from tiring yourself out).

Without anaesthesia, most women don't need to be taught how to push – it's an irresistible urge. However, if you've received pain relief, in particular an epidural, you may be too numb to feel the contractions, in which case you may need some coaching by your doctor or midwife. In some cases, the dose of the epidural will need to be lowered or turned off entirely in order to allow some sensation to return. Once the baby begins to crown, many women also experience a fierce burning sensation as the baby stretches out the skin of the perineum, often referred to as the 'ring of fire'. This can be excruciating, but is usually (mercifully) brief, giving the tissue a chance to stretch adequately and helping to prevent perineal tears and lacerations.

Finding a good position

You can push in any number of positions, although many hospitals will want you to remain in bed during this phase. If you do have to stay in the bed, try to push in a position which allows you to take advantage of the natural benefits of gravity. Most hospital beds can accommodate a variety of positions, though, and you may find that pushing while lying on your side or sitting is more comfortable. Some hospital beds are even equipped with a bar which you can hold on to while squatting, which is a great position for opening your pelvis and giving your baby more room to descend.

Many women find pushing on hands and knees, squatting, kneeling, standing or leaning on someone or something to be ideal. Pushing in a waterbirth pool is also a great option if it's available, with the added benefit that the water pressure helps the skin of the perineum to stretch. The position for birth is based on several factors: your own personal comfort, how effectively you're pushing, the size or position of the baby and the comfort and experience of the person performing the delivery. In general, though, gravity is your best friend; upright positions will help the baby deliver more quickly, and often gives the pelvis more room to stretch and open up.

Condensed idea
Pushing marks the beginning of the end of labour

The doc steps in

Most women have an uncomplicated labour and don't need much assistance. However, if a complication does arise, labour can be induced, slowed down or accelerated; vacuum or forceps can help tricky deliveries; and caesarean sections are available for emergencies.

Inducing labour

'Induction' is the use of drugs to make labour begin, rather than allowing it to start naturally. There are a lot of reasons why your doctor or midwife might suggest this as an option, including maternal reasons (such as pre-eclampsia), foetal reasons (such as low amniotic fluid), premature rupture of membranes (you may be allowed 12–24 hours to go into natural labour if this happens, unless there's reason to act immediately), or an overdue pregnancy.

> Jamie got his head stuck but the doc soon helped him out. Hurray for the vacuum thingy. #sorelieved

The first phase of an induction usually involves administering a cervical-ripening agent to soften and prepare your cervix, followed by synthetic oxytocin to begin contractions. In general, induction can be a very long process; sometimes it can take one to two days of cervical ripening before the oxytocin is given. Inductions have a slightly higher chance of resulting in a caesarean, but most are successful if given enough time. If they're done for a medical reason (as opposed to convenience), the benefits of the induction outweigh the risks.

Augmenting labour

Unlike induction, augmentation occurs after labour has already started on its own. In many cases, it's used to increase the adequacy of contractions if no progress is being made (i.e. creating contractions strong enough to dilate and efface the cervix). Natural ways to augment labour include walking, starting an IV drip to help combat dehydration, or 'sweeping the membranes'. This is done by your midwife or doctor during a vaginal exam – she stretches the cervix and gently separates the membranes from the cervical opening with her finger. She may also break the bag of waters (this is known as amniotomy). However, most often women are given synthetic oxytocin if they need help in strengthening the rate and intensity of contractions. This is always administered intravenously and is very carefully controlled, so as not to over-stimulate the uterus and cause foetal stress and exhaustion. It is always accompanied by continuous electronic foetal monitoring.

Assisted delivery

In 10–15 per cent of all births, forceps or a vacuum (ventouse) is used to help assist with the delivery of the baby's head. This tends to happen after a long, protracted labour, when the woman is exhausted and struggling to actually push the baby out, or if there is evidence of foetal distress. In both cases, the head is usually already quite low in the pelvis, often visible, and the forceps or vacuum are used to help pull the baby's head down the last few inches in concert with the woman's pushing efforts.

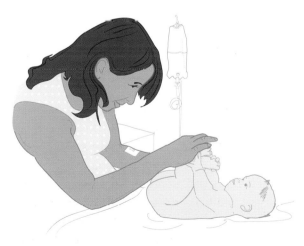

Assisted delivery with vacuum or forceps is almost always done by a doctor rather than a midwife, and may require anaesthesia for pain relief and an episiotomy (see box below for more information) to help widen the opening of the vagina. These days vacuum is used much more frequently than forceps because the parts in contact with the baby are softer and more flexible. In some cases, forceps or vacuum use can increase the risk of vaginal lacerations, as well as occasionally bruising the baby's scalp or (very rarely) injuring the infant in some way. With most assisted deliveries, though, only a few extra pulls are needed to bring the baby's head down to the point of crowning, at which point the woman can usually take over, pushing the baby out naturally.

What they don't tell you...

Many women dread the thought of an episiotomy (an incision made at the outlet of the vagina to help open the soft tissue) and some find even the word disquieting. Around 25 years ago, episiotomies were performed routinely at nearly every vaginal delivery, but we've learned a lot since then about how the perineum stretches, tears and recovers. Most naturally occurring lacerations are very superficial, and even though they can be more irregular and jagged than a neat, surgical episiotomy, they tend to heal more quickly. An episiotomy is a deep-muscle cut that is generally used as a measure of last resort, in emergencies when the baby needs to get out very quickly or during a vacuum or forceps delivery. These days performing an episiotomy on the vaginal tissue is a very rare occurrence, but it doesn't hurt to ask about your healthcare provider's views on it well before you're actually pushing.

Caesareans

Caesareans are carried out for a variety of reasons. In some cases, it's scheduled before you even go into labour – perhaps you have had a caesarean before or your baby is in a breech position. In other cases, the decision is made during labour due to foetal distress, a baby not descending, or a cervix that won't dilate after hours and hours of trying. The decision to operate should never be made lightly – a caesarean is major abdominal surgery requiring weeks of convalescence afterwards, with much higher risks of infection, blood loss and complications than vaginal delivery. If you've already had one caesarean, you might want to research the possibility of having a VBAC (vaginal birth after caesarean) for your next pregnancy.

During a caesarean, an anaesthetist uses an epidural or spinal injection to make you numb from the breasts down. Sterile drapes are then applied to your abdomen, and your belly and the surgical site are carefully cleaned. Most often a low incision is made above your hips, commonly referred to as a 'bikini cut', and the baby is delivered through the incision. Afterwards, the incision is repaired. In rare cases, general anaesthesia is used rather than epidural anaesthesia.

As with assisted deliveries, caesareans are performed by doctors only, although your midwife may come with you into the operating room and assist. Afterwards you are taken to a recovery room where your vital signs and urine output are very carefully monitored for several hours. Many hospitals are now becoming much more family-friendly during caesareans, often allowing a partner or family member to accompany a pregnant woman into the operating room.

Condensed idea
Sometimes a little extra help is needed but it's no cause for alarm

You did it!

At last, your baby has arrived. How magical and emotional those first moments are, as you look at your newborn for the very first time. Even though it might feel like all the hard work is done, the labour isn't quite over – there's still the third and fourth stage to get through.

Savour the moment

No matter what has yet to happen, take a moment to stop, breathe deeply and revel in the moment. You just gave birth! If there are no issues with your newborn requiring extra care or resuscitation, she will probably be placed in your arms immediately after the delivery. Soak her up! Gaze in wonder at her tiny perfection, count her fingers and toes, marvel over her little face, which will probably be staring right at you and talk soothingly to her – she will undoubtedly recognize and be comforted by your voice. Nestle her against your skin and enjoy. This is what all of the hard work was for.

Delivering the placenta

While you're bonding with your newborn, your midwife or doctor will be waiting for signs of placental separation. Now that the baby is delivered, the uterus is quickly shrinking and contracting, and the placenta begins to detach from the uterine wall. Signs include a small gush of blood and lengthening of the cord, and you may feel a few deep cramps in the uterus – although nothing like the painful contractions of active labour.

Your doctor or midwife will deliver the placenta by gently drawing it downward by the cord, and will usually ask you to help with the delivery

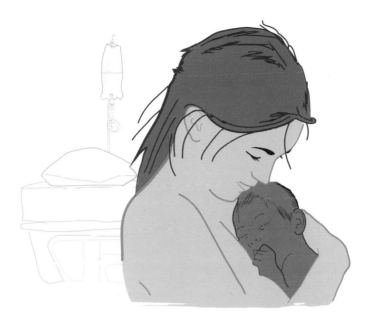

by giving a few mild pushes. Delivering the placenta is normally
painless. It takes anywhere from a few minutes to an hour for the
placenta to separate, and there's no harm in waiting as long as you're
not actively bleeding. If for some reason your placenta still hasn't been
delivered after an hour (a phenomenon known as a 'retained placenta'),
steps may need to be taken to encourage it to separate. You may be
asked to squat or to nurse the baby, which releases more oxytocin and
helps the uterus contract. If you have a full bladder getting in the way
of the placenta, you will be asked to urinate, or a catheter may be used
to drain your bladder. Finally, if none of these tricks work, your midwife
or doctor may have to manually remove the placenta with their hand,
usually done under anaesthesia.

The fourth, final stage

Once the placenta is out, the fourth stage of labour begins. This is known
as the recovery phase. While it might seem like everything is finished,
your body is going through huge adjustments as it makes the transition

from pregnant to not-pregnant, and your doctor or midwife will want to keep a close eye on you. Many women experience shaking and teeth-chattering during this time, which is normal, and warm blankets usually help. Your vital signs and bleeding will be very closely monitored, and your uterus will be checked to make sure it is tightly contracted, clamping down on the blood vessels left open after the separation of the placenta.

> I get to hold baby John while Anna gets a good checking over. So relieved to know that both of them are fine. #newborndad

If you have a laceration or have been given an episiotomy, your doctor or midwife will do the repair at this time, using a local anaesthetic. The good news is that the perineum is one of the most forgiving parts of the body: it heals incredibly quickly, and within six weeks most women won't even be able to see a scar (you can read more about this on pages 184–87). The recovery phase is also the perfect time to begin breastfeeding (see pages 176–79).

Cord-blood banking

Cord-blood banking has recently gained a great deal of popularity. The idea behind it is that by saving the stem cells found in the cord blood, these may be used at a later point to treat disease in any member of the family. However, while stem cells are already being used to treat a variety of diseases, such as leukaemia, if your family doesn't currently suffer from one of these diseases, the chance of developing one and needing the stem cells is 1 in 10,000. Nevertheless, some families still choose to save and bank the blood on the chance that future research will reveal new applications for stem cells. Before the placenta is delivered, the blood is collected painlessly from the umbilical cord by your healthcare provider after the cord has been cut (so it doesn't affect the baby in any way).

Postnatal warning signs

While most women sail smoothly and easily through the initial postnatal period, be on the lookout for any of the following signs, and let your nurse, midwife or doctor know right away if you notice any of them.

- Heavy bleeding: soaking more than two maternity pads in one hour or less, or bleeding which is increasing rather than decreasing.
- Passing blood clots larger than the size of a 10 pence coin.
- Any foul-smelling vaginal discharge, or any discharge that's green or yellow.
- Any fever higher than 38°C (100.4°F).
- Shaking or chills.
- Abdominal pain, particularly if you had a caesarean.
- Severe pain in the perineum: any pain that is so severe that you have difficulty walking, or pain which increases over time.
- Pain, tenderness, swelling, warmth or redness in the breasts, legs or calves.
- Warmth, spreading redness, or yellow or green discharge from your incision site if you had a caesarean.

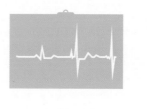

Condensed idea
The hard work is done, but the process isn't considered finished until one hour after the delivery

41 The best-laid plans...

It's impossible to avoid having expectations for your birth, but unfortunately, it's not something you have total control over and sometimes the birth is very different to the one you hoped for. If this happens to you, try to focus on the outcome, not the process.

Being flexible in every way

Once you've been through labour and given birth, you'll probably realize why people say that the greatest gift you can give to yourself during the process is a flexible attitude. Over the course of the pregnancy and then right through labour, your body will have shown its own incredible flexibility, and you need to allow your mind to demonstrate a similar willingness to accept and deal with whatever happens. Because no matter how many births you see or hear about before your own experience of it,

> Everything was different to how I expected but who cares? He's beautiful. #contentmum

and however many careful decisions you make on your birth plan, the chances are that the birth will probably turn out completely differently to your expectations. This doesn't mean that there's no point in preparing – taking childbirth classes, learning natural pain coping techniques, and finding a caring provider who shares your birth philosophy are all vitally important to helping ensure a safe and satisfying birth experience. But on top of all of this, it's important to cultivate a 'go-with-the-flow' attitude and cut yourself some slack. You can't control your birth, but you can control how you react to whatever your labour throws at you.

If you're reading this before you give birth, spend some time considering each of the ways you might deliver your baby. Even if you have your heart set on a home birth, for instance, spend some time thinking about what you would do if you needed to give birth via caesarean, and how you would welcome your baby in an operating room rather than your living room. If you're planning on having an epidural, picture yourself getting to the hospital hoping for immediate pain relief, only to discover that you're almost fully dilated and there isn't time. It's impossible to run through every potential birth scenario, but doing this exercise helps remind you that there are plenty of alternatives to whatever you're hoping for, and that none of them are bad options – they're just different.

After you've considered the various options, do something that might seem bizarre – let them go. Now just try to prepare yourself for whatever might come. There are larger forces at work during the birth than just you alone. Your baby, for instance, might have plans of his own, and depending on what happens, various interventions may be required to help him. Or you may require special interventions that you hadn't considered, such as an induction, rather than the natural labour you'd been planning on. The most important outcome of all is a healthy mum and a healthy baby. It helps to put that at the forefront of your mind, and consider everything else along the way as simply the story of your childbirth, which will be unique, unpredictable and wholly yours.

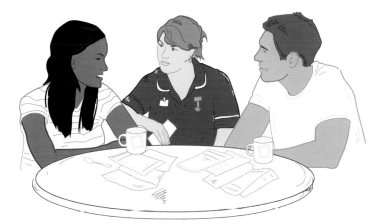

If the birth went 'wrong'…

We discussed the use of sentence-stemming on page 15 as a technique for emotional release. If you find yourself disappointed by the birth and unable to let it go, try writing down as many endings as you can think of to the following sentences:

- When I think about my birth, I am most disappointed by…
- If I could do it over again, I would…
- The thing about my birth I most need to keep in mind is…
- When I think about my birth, I am thankful for…
- If I could tell someone else about my birth, I would say…
- The worst thing about my birth was…
- The best thing about my birth was…

Don't beat yourself up

If, for whatever reason, your birth does not go according to plan and you find yourself upset by this, it's crucial to acknowledge and express this disappointment in order to heal. If you keep your feelings to yourself and quietly beat yourself up about it, it will forever be an issue that you'll carry around with you. Be compassionate with yourself, especially in the challenging and emotional weeks immediately after the delivery, when you'll be tender, sensitive and exhausted. The very first things to banish are any feelings of guilt or failure – if things didn't go according to plan, this certainly wasn't because of something you did or did not do. Nevertheless, it's important to recognize that whatever you're feeling is perfectly real and valid.

Disappointment over the birth is a type of loss (the loss of the dream you had for your birth), and must pass through the five stages of grief – denial, anger, bargaining, depression and acceptance – before finally healing. Time is your biggest ally in this, but it will also help to talk to a friend or therapist, lean on your support network, or use meditation, yoga, birth regression or art therapy to help you work through what has happened. Going over your birth story with your midwife or doctor might also help you understand what happened and why, and would give you a chance to voice your concerns and regrets. You may also find it helpful to write about your birth story in a journal. Midwife Pam England suggests exploring the power of our unconscious mind through the use of art. This is a great tool to help you realize what your deep-seated fears and concerns are during pregnancy, and it can also serve as an excellent way to heal yourself afterwards.

Look for the gift

One of the best ways of getting over a huge disappointment is to look at the positive aspects that have arisen from the experience. For example, if your care provider hadn't insisted that you go straight to the hospital, despite your insistence that you wanted a home birth, there's a strong chance that you or your baby would have suffered from serious complications. Or, if you ended up having a caesarean after dreaming only of having a natural birth, perhaps you could dwell on the fact that you gave your partner the wonderful gift of being the first person to hold the baby. Whatever may have gone 'wrong' in your eyes, just remember that the most important thing is that incredible bundle of joy that you miraculously created and get to keep, no matter how he ended up arriving into this world!

Condensed idea
Giving birth requires a great deal of flexibility in mind and body

42 The golden hour

The first hour after birth, commonly referred to as the golden hour, is perhaps the most important hour of your baby's life. He or she is making a huge transition from intrauterine to extrauterine life, and now is the most important time to bond with your brand new child.

Hello world!

Imagine birth from your baby's point of view: suddenly thrust out of the warm, quiet, familiar darkness of the womb into the cold, bright, noisy, over-stimulating world, where he doesn't recognize anything and has lost both your heartbeat and your voice, which have been the background noise of his entire existence. You can make a huge difference by using the first hour after her birth to help him during this transition; your gentle comfort now will help calm and relax him, stabilize his vital signs and teach him that he's not alone.

If there are no complications that necessitate additional care for your baby, request that he be placed immediately on your chest after the delivery. This is the safest and most reassuring place for him to be, and there are countless benefits of skin-to-skin bonding: you baby will be warmer and calmer; he can hear your heartbeat through your chest; his heart rate, temperature and breathing rate will normalize; and your milk supply

> I can finally touch him, after all those months of waiting. He even seemed to know my voice. #lovingmum

To clamp or not to clamp?

In addition to delaying non-medical procedures such as weighing and measuring the baby during the first hour, you might like to find out whether your hospital is willing to delay clamping the umbilical cord until the cord has stopped pulsing. Substantial amounts of research have shown that delaying clamping by even one or two minutes can make a big difference. Here are just a few of the benefits of waiting to cut the cord:

- Babies with delayed cord clamping have 32 per cent more blood volume than babies whose cords are clamped immediately after delivery.
- Increased blood volume leads to higher levels of stored iron and a two-minute delay in cord clamping improves the iron status of babies for up to six months after birth.
- Babies with their full blood volume are able to transition more easily to life outside the womb.
- Delayed cord clamping offers protection from brain haemorrhage and improves outcomes in premature infants.

will improve, making breastfeeding easier when the time comes. During labour, your body generates hormones which prime you for bonding, even going so far as changing your brain chemistry to increase your desire for nurturing. Direct skin-to-skin contact with your baby after the birth is what cements these changes in place, releasing the nurturing hormone oxytocin and forming the basis of your attachment to your baby. It also helps contract the uterus, prevent haemorrhage, and improves the chances of your baby's wellbeing, as well as promoting long-term breastfeeding success.

Nine stages of transition

Research has shown that babies placed on their mother's chest immediately after delivery go through nine instinctive stages. The very first stage is the birth cry, which helps the baby clear the fluid in his lungs, followed by a period of relaxation where he might rest on your chest covered by a warm blanket, without much movement or crying. After the relaxation stage, the baby then awakens again and begins to move his head and shoulders, opens his eyes and exhibits some mouth movement – this stage usually starts about three minutes after the birth.

The next stage is a period of activity where the newborn begins to make more mouthing and sucking movements, and may begin to root at the breast by moving his mouth from side to side. The baby may go through another stage of rest after this, but eventually, if left on his own, the baby will begin to 'crawl' towards the breast, usually accomplished by wiggling, lunging, rooting and sliding. Eventually, once the baby has found the breast, he will go through a stage of familiarization, where he becomes acquainted with you and may lick, nuzzle and knead your breast, as well as looking at you and making soft sounds to get your attention (this licking and kneading does more to promote milk production and let-down than the actual sucking itself, amazingly). Finally, he will attach himself to a nipple and begin to suck; if left on his own, this is usually accomplished by the end of the first hour after birth.

Making the most of your hour

Just a few short years ago, the first hour after birth was owned by the medical profession. Babies were delivered and handed to a nurse, who would then take the baby to a warmer, weigh and measure him, inject vitamin K, apply eye ointment and finally (finally!) wrap the baby up and hand him back to the waiting parents. These days, most hospitals aim to put the baby into the mother's arms for the first hour of life, but check beforehand whether this is standard practice for your hospital.

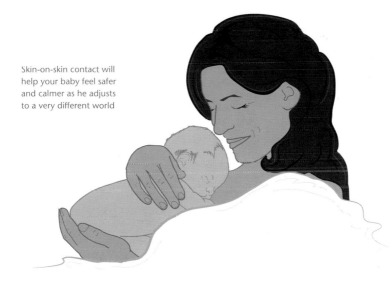

Skin-on-skin contact will help your baby feel safer and calmer as he adjusts to a very different world

If for some reason a medical condition requires that your baby be stabilized and taken to intensive care immediately after the delivery, or if you give birth via caesarean and aren't able to hold your baby right away, the golden hour becomes the very first hour that the two of you are reunited and you're able to hold him for the first time. If it's impossible to hold your baby, you can simulate the golden hour by touching him, getting as close to him as possible so that he can smell your scent, and talking softly to him – your familiar voice will help soothe and calm him. Research has shown the many benefits of skin-to-skin contact to premature babies or those in intensive care. The staff may have to help transfer the baby to your chest, especially if there are tubes or wires attached, but your baby will still benefit tremendously from close contact with you. So say hello, whatever the conditions.

Condensed idea
The first hour of life offers a unique opportunity for you to bond with your baby

43 Checking baby

After some bonding, snuggling and breastfeeding, it's time to examine your brand new baby and make sure everything is fine. The all-important weight and height will be measured by your midwife or doctor, and some of this can be done while the baby remains in your arms.

Instant Apgar test

The Apgar score is a way of evaluating a baby's condition at birth based on a scoring system developed by Dr Virginia Apgar in the 1950s. The Apgar score looks at five key elements (colour, muscle tone, heart rate, respiratory rate and cry) at the time of delivery, and again five minutes after the birth, as a way of assessing how well the newborn is adapting to life outside the womb. A score of 2 is given to each element if the baby is pink, vigorous and crying, with a normal heart rate and respiratory rate. A score of 1 or zero is given if the baby doesn't meet the criteria for each element. A low Apgar score may mean that the baby needs additional help, such as oxygen, suctioning or positive pressure ventilation. If the baby is transitioning well, a total score of 9 or 10 is usually the norm.

The initial assessment

The initial assessment may be done at the bedside, with the baby in your arms, or at the warmer. In some hospitals it doesn't happen until the baby is taken to the newborn nursery, while in other hospitals the baby may be kept with you all the time. If your baby does go to the nursery, your partner or another family member may be able to accompany her. Your baby may also be identified with a bracelet at ankle and wrist before going to the nursery, and in some countries footprints or handprints are taken.

A paediatrician or midwife will unwrap the baby and examine all parts of her. Her head will be checked for any swelling, cuts or bruises known as cephalohaematomas, which may last for several weeks or even a few months before spontaneously resolving. Sometimes the baby's head has been squashed into a cone shape during birth (known as 'moulding') but this usually disappears within 24–48 hours. The baby's skin will be inspected for any rashes or birthmarks such as Mongolian spots (dark

The circumcision decision

Certain religions have been practising circumcision for centuries, but routine circumcision didn't become popular in the USA until the late 1800s, under the belief that circumcision would prevent masturbation (it doesn't). Today approximately 63 per cent of all boys in the USA are still circumcised, often due to concerns over cleanliness, to spare the boy ridicule from his peers, or so that the son's penis looks like his father's.

However, in Europe and the rest of the world, circumcision for non-religious or medical reasons remains extremely rare. While some research has shown that circumcision may lower the rates of urinary tract infections and penile cancer in boys and men, the benefit gained by this practice is marginal since the incidence of both of these is very low. Circumcision is a painful procedure (the pain can be lessened slightly by various forms of anaesthesia) and carries risks of blood loss, injury and infection. Opponents also argue that the procedure to remove a functioning part of the baby's body is done without the baby's consent. The decision to circumcise is a complex and very personal choice, which should be researched carefully.

blue-black pigmented areas on the low back or buttocks, which are harmless and usually fade within a few years) or stork marks (small, flat red marks caused by broken capillaries in the skin which usually fade within a few weeks). Your healthcare provider will examine your baby's eyes, listen to the heart and lungs, check the spine to make sure it is straight and check the baby's hips for hip dysplasia (where one of the femur bones is not properly aligned in the hip socket).

A quick assessment will be done of your baby's reflexes, including her startle reflex (known as the Moro reflex), which happens when the baby hears a loud sound or experiences a sudden movement – she will fling up her arms with her hands in a C-shape, throw back her head, extend her legs, and then pull her arms and legs back in again. Other reflexes like the sucking and rooting reflex, the grasping reflex and the stepping reflex will also be tested. Normal reflex response demonstrates the presence of an intact nervous system and normal brain activity.

Your baby will also probably receive an injection of vitamin K at this time to ensure proper blood clotting. Vitamin K is normally synthesized by bacteria in our colons, but when babies are born they lack these

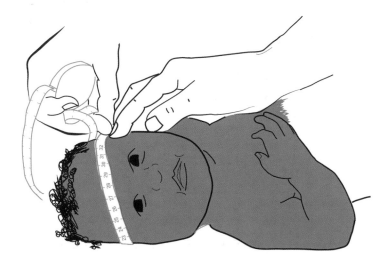

necessary bacteria (although they quickly gain them over the next few weeks, especially if breastfeeding), which is why the injection is needed. If you object to your baby having an injection, it's possible to give oral drops instead, but it's harder to ensure that the baby is getting the correct dose using this method.

Finally, the baby will be weighed and measured so that her growth rate can be tracked over the next several weeks and months. On average, babies weigh 2.6–4 kg (6–9 lb) and are around 50 cm (20 in) long. Most babies lose up to 10 per cent of their initial birth weight within a week of birth. Breastfed

> Baby lost a point on the Apgar cos his feet were bluish. Otherwise perfect (9/10). #competingalready

babies tend to lose a bit more than formula-fed babies, but this is normal and expected. Most babies regain their birth weight by the time they are around 10–14 days old.

Newborn screening

In most countries, infants receive a blood test that screens for several genetic diseases and congenital errors in metabolism, because prompt diagnosis and treatment can help avoid developmental delays or even death. The test involves taking a sample of blood from your baby's heel, sometimes causing the heel to bruise or remain red for a few days. Breastfeeding your baby immediately afterwards will help diminish the pain and provide much-needed comfort.

Condensed idea
Rest assured that your baby will be thoroughly checked for any health problems soon after the birth

(44) Breasts and bottles

There is no doubt that breastfeeding is the healthiest option available for your baby. While in some rare cases formula may be necessary, try to establish breastfeeding if at all possible, because this is a gift that only you can give to your baby.

Why breast is best

Breastfeeding is better for you and your baby in every regard. Breast milk is uniquely designed to be perfectly absorbed by your baby, and will provide all of her nutritional needs for the first six months of her life. Milk formulas for bottle feeding can mimic a few of the nutritional components of breast milk, but not all. Breastfeeding also helps your body adapt and recover.

The composition of breast milk changes on a daily basis, giving your baby more of what she needs for each stage of her growth. No formula can match this custom-made, easily digestible food. Breast milk also helps prevent infections in your baby by providing antibacterial and antiviral agents, passing on your own immune antibodies to help passively guard your infant from disease, and stimulating your infant's own immune system as well. Babies who breastfeed have lower rates of allergies, rashes, ear infections, eczema and asthma. Breast milk has also been shown to prevent illnesses in your child – such as Crohn's disease, lymphoma and even diabetes – when she's much older.

> So glad the midwife helped me work out this breastfeeding thing. Not so hard after all! #nursingmum

Breastfeeding has many benefits for you as well. In the first few days after the birth, breastfeeding helps contract the uterus and prevent heavy bleeding. It also speeds up your metabolism, so you will lose any extra pregnancy weight more quickly. Research even suggests that breastfeeding may help protect the mother against breast cancer and ovarian cancer. It's also incredibly rewarding, providing a special bond between you and your baby. And of course, don't forget the convenience – breastfeeding is absolutely free and much easier to do in the middle of the night, as there are no bottles to sterilize or formula to warm and prepare.

Getting started

Breastfeeding needs very little advance preparation. There is no need to toughen up or prepare your nipples in any way for nursing, and in fact, excessive stimulation of the nipples during pregnancy may cause premature contractions. Ideally, breastfeeding will begin during the golden hour (see pages 168–71) right after birth. However, even if you're

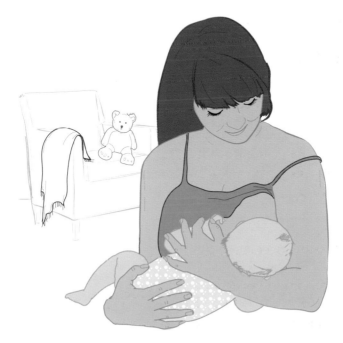

unable to nurse right away, it's still possible to get off to a great start – it just might take a little more work. Your nurse, midwife or even a lactation consultant can help position your baby and assist with latching.

Your initial milk is known as colostrum, which is a very nutrient-rich blend full of antibodies, with the consistency of honey. Even though it's hard to

It's all about the latch

Establishing a good latch at the breast is one of the best ways to ensure that your baby is getting enough milk, as well as preventing sore and cracked nipples, so try the following steps:

- Sit back comfortably – bring the baby to you, rather than the other way around. Try propping nursing pillows under your arms and the baby to make nursing more comfortable.
- Support your breast with one hand, and place the baby's mouth within easy reach of your nipple.
- Make sure the baby's face and body are turned in towards you.
- Tickle the baby's lips with the nipple and wait for her to open her mouth.
- Once she's opening wide (it looks like a yawn), bring the nipple into her mouth, with her head tipped back slightly and her chin pressing into the breast.
- The baby's suck stimulus is on the roof of the mouth towards the back of the palate. Once the baby feels the nipple there, she will close her mouth and begin to suck.
- A good latch will feel like a strong tug, but not pinching and painful. If it hurts, unlatch the baby by putting a finger in her mouth to break the seal, and try again.

see evidence of milk in the first few days and it may seem as though your baby wants to nurse constantly (on average, 10–12 times in the first 24 hours), you'll produce enough – your baby only needs a tablespoon or two at each feeding. Within two to three days, your milk will begin to come in, and your breasts may become engorged and tender. It's very important to continue to nurse during this time, as this helps to establish your milk supply as well as helping to ease the engorgement. You'll know your baby is getting enough when you see 2–3 stools a day and 5–6 wet nappies a day by day 3–4. The baby will also have good colour and skin tone, be growing and filling out, and satisfied after a feeding.

Bottlefeeding basics

If you're unable to breastfeed, there are several formulas available which your baby can drink instead. Made from cow or soya milk, they are all more difficult to digest than breast milk, which helps explain why formula-fed babies tend to stay full for longer – it takes their bodies longer to process their meal.

Commercial formulas can be bought in liquid and powder form. There is an abundance of bottles and teats on the market, many designed to mimic real nipples or prevent air and gas bubbles from entering the baby – experiment with a few different brands to see what your baby prefers. All bottles should be sterilized before use; this helps prevent germs or bacteria from the water supply infecting your baby's immature immune system. Never use a microwave to heat the bottle, as this creates hot pockets which can scald the baby. And remember, bottle-fed babies deserve to be snuggled skin to skin while feeding too!

Condensed idea
Your body knew just how to grow a baby, and now it knows how to feed her perfectly too

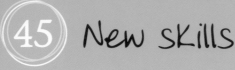

45 New skills

The first few weeks with a new baby can seem a bit daunting. It's comforting to know that what your baby wants more than anything else is to be with you. The rest will come with practice, and you'll be amazed at how quickly you gain confidence in your new parenting skills.

Nappy changing

For the first few days your baby's stool is a very dark, sticky tar-like substance known as meconium. This is basically all of the amniotic fluid the baby has been swallowing during the pregnancy, digested and expelled. After two to three days, as your milk begins to come in, the baby's stool begins to have a dark green appearance, which is perfectly normal. By day four or five, it should start to look yellow or mustard-coloured, and is usually soft and runny (although occasionally it can look seedy or grainy, caused by milk curds). If you notice any blood in the stool, or anything which looks like dark coffee grounds (dried blood), contact your doctor immediately. However, the baby's urine in the first two days can sometimes have an orange, red or rust-coloured appearance caused by urea crystals, which is normal and shouldn't be confused with blood.

Whatever type of nappy you're using, putting on the very first one can be a challenge, but you'll very quickly learn to manoeuvre your squirming little baby and get the job done. Nappy rash caused by moisture and skin irritation is incredibly common. Nappy creams can help, but one of the best cures is to ditch the nappy for a few hours and let everything air out a bit. You can place your baby on an old towel, blanket or cloth during this time to prevent accidents.

When to call the doc

Never feel guilty about calling the doctor for reassurance or support. It's much better to be safe than sorry. Call your doctor promptly if you notice any of the following:

- A temperature higher than 38°C (100.4°F).
- Your baby is listless or behaving strangely (seems 'not himself').
- If your baby hasn't had a bowel movement for 48 hours.
- If your baby doesn't urinate within the first 24 hours of life (this only applies if you've had a home birth; in a hospital, the staff will be keeping tabs on this).
- If you notice wheezing, grunting or whistling sounds during breathing.
- If you notice any retracting (pulling in of the ribs) as your baby breathes in and out.
- If the baby's eyes or skin look yellow (it might be easier to check in natural light; blanch the skin by pressing firmly on it then releasing – the skin will look yellow when you take your finger away).
- If you notice any oozing of pus or a foul odour or discharge around the cord stump.

Cord care

The umbilical cord stump usually dries out and falls off around 5–6 days after the birth, but can sometimes take up to a week or more after the delivery. At no point should you try to remove the stump manually, or pick at it – it will simply fall off on its own when it's ready. While the stump is still attached, soak a cotton swab or cotton-wool bud in surgical spirit and very gently clean around the base of the stump, at the point that it meets the skin. This helps prevent infections and encourages the stump to dry out more quickly. Most newborn nappies have a cut-out in the front to prevent the nappy from rubbing against the cord, but if the brand you're using doesn't, simply fold the top down slightly so it doesn't touch the cord stump.

Swaddle for security

For the first few weeks, your baby will be happiest if he's tightly wrapped in a swaddle, which mimics the close quarters of the womb and helps him to feel at home. His new freedom of movement and lack of control over his limbs at this stage means that he's likely to inadvertently whack himself in the face from time to time, so the tight confines of a swaddle are reassuring for that reason as well. There are plenty of demonstrations online, or you can ask your midwife or nurse to show you how to swaddle your baby.

Bathtime

For the first few days, while the cord stump is still attached, it's best just to wipe your baby down with a warm, wet sponge while he's lying on a towel. When you're ready for your first baby bath, gather everything you'll need close at hand before you start: a hooded towel, a flannel or sponge, some baby soap, a clean nappy and change of clothes. It might also help to heat the room slightly before the bath. The water should be at room temperature – test it on your inner arm to make sure it's not too hot. There are plenty of bath thermometers on the market that are specially designed to go in the water to test the temperature before you put the baby in.

> Finally brave enough to give her a proper bath. No damage done. In fact I think she quite liked it! #soggymum

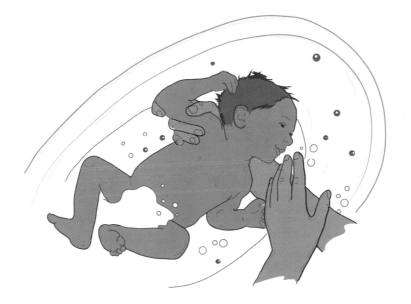

Begin with the baby's face, using a clean flannel or sponge without soap. Wipe his eyes with two separate, clean and dampened pieces of cotton wool – this avoids any danger of eye infection. Use the sponge or flannel to clean behind the ears, then gently work your way downwards, bathing the baby's trunk, back, armpits, groin area and finally legs and feet. Rinse with the flannel, sponge, or a cup of water. When you pour water over the baby's head, tip him backwards so that the water doesn't fall into his eyes. Newborns don't actually get that dirty and soap can dry out their skin, so using just water in the beginning is better. You don't need to fully bathe them every day, but a small sponge bath of the groin area daily is recommended. And remember: never leave your baby unattended in the bath.

Condensed idea
Taking care of a newborn can be stressful – but in a couple of weeks your parenting skills will shine

46 Newborn mum

It's easy for your own needs to get lost in the activity surrounding a newborn, but as you're still recovering from the birth, you need to take good care of yourself. You will adjust more easily if others are available to nurture you, so that you can nurture the baby.

Helping the healing

It's normal to feel incredibly sore and tender for several weeks after a delivery, particularly if you had an episiotomy or laceration. As discussed earlier (see page 158), thanks to the excellent blood flow this part of your body usually heals very quickly, and any stitches are absorbed directly by your body. However, a few small steps can help soothe the tender tissue and promote healing. In some countries an ice pack is sometimes placed on the perineum for the first 24 hours after the delivery, to help reduce inflammation and ease the pain. After that, warm soaks work better to promote healing than ice. Some hospitals have sitz baths: small plastic baths which fit into the toilet seat to allow you to soak your perineum in warm water several times a day. You can purchase one for yourself if you have a home birth. Some healthcare providers recommend adding Epsom salts or a combination of herbs to the water to promote healing (lavender, uva ursi, sage and witch hazel are all good choices). It's also helpful to use a small squirt bottle to rinse yourself with water rather than wiping with toilet paper after urination; this helps

> The park is full of new mums walking about. I made three new friends just this morning!
> #healingmum

Renewing intimacy

There is no hard and fast rule on when you
can resume sex after delivery. If the bright red
bleeding has stopped and you don't notice any
pain, it's safe to have sex, but let your body
be your guide. You may find yourself raring
to go in only a few weeks, or needing to wait
six months or more before you feel physically
and emotionally ready. So much is going on
in the first few months that (unsurprisingly)
sex is usually put on a back-burner for a
while. For many women, there is still lingering
physical pain, combined with sleep deprivation, postnatal blues,
breastfeeding on demand, body image issues arising from
pregnancy weight or stretch marks, plus the huge adjustment
to new family roles. Even so, you and your partner still need
love, affirmation and affection, so be sure to keep those lines of
communication open. If sex is not an option initially, make time for
cuddles, kissing, spooning, massages and affectionate touch. And
when the moment does arrive (whenever that may be), go slow
and be compassionate and tender with yourself and your partner.

avoid scratching or aggravating the tissue. After a bowel movement, you
can also rinse yourself with warm, soapy water rather than wipe, and
then pat yourself dry afterwards. Pads or compresses soaked in witch hazel
and applied directly to your perineum, or laid on top of your maternity
pads, also feel heavenly – even more so if they've been kept in the fridge
so that they're nice and cold before applying. In some cases, your midwife
or doctor may prescribe a topical anaesthetic cream or spray which helps
relieve the pain.

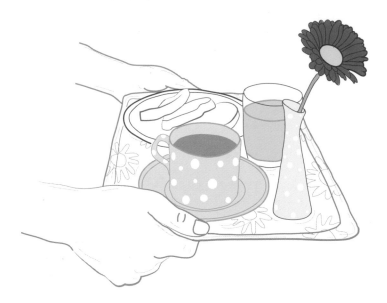

You'll experience some bleeding, known as lochia, for around three to four weeks after the birth. For the first few days, the lochia is bright red, like a menstrual period. Then it becomes progressively lighter in colour until it finally disappears. Occasionally, if you're trying to do too much too soon, the flow may become darker and heavier again. This is a signal to put your feet up and truly rest for a day or two, which should correct it. However, if you notice heavy, bright red bleeding 4–8 weeks after you gave birth, don't panic – it's just your period, which you haven't seen in quite a while. This may return as early as four weeks or as late as a year or more, depending on whether you're exclusively breastfeeding or not.

Weight and exercise

You will miraculously lose about 5.5–6.5 kg (12–14 lb) after the delivery, just by giving birth. As you begin to breastfeed, your metabolism will also begin to speed up, which helps hasten the process. About 37 per cent of women return to their pre-pregnancy weight six months after the birth. Most women who had an uncomplicated vaginal delivery can begin exercising again as soon as the lochia has disappeared, but if you had a caesarean, it's a good idea to wait a bit longer, until at least six weeks after the birth. In either case, take it easy – most personal trainers recommend spending several weeks doing nothing more arduous than walking. Keep yourself well hydrated while exercising, and stop before you feel tired. Above all, be gentle with yourself and remember that your body needs time to readjust.

Ups and downs

Be prepared for a few emotional weeks right after the birth. While the first few days can be spent in a haze of excitement, it doesn't take long for the exhaustion of your new role to catch up with you. Coupled with the normal hormonal changes occurring as your body makes the transition from pregnant to not-pregnant, most women find themselves on a bit of an emotional rollercoaster.

You may find yourself feeling invincible one moment, then crying for no good reason the next, or confronted by feelings of doubt, ambivalence and negativity at odd moments, which can sometimes seem very incongruous in the face of such a happy event. However, all of these feelings are incredibly normal and common, and usually go away on their own after a week or so (if they don't, you might be experiencing postnatal depression, which will be covered in more detail on pages 196–99). Don't be scared to talk about your feelings – expressing your emotions, even the negative ones, will help you process them. The best medicine is meeting with other brand new mums and hearing from them that you're not alone.

Condensed idea
The month after the birth is a time of huge adjustment for you in mind and body

47 The first few weeks

Early days with a new baby can be absolutely gruelling, but keep your chin up: they're short-lived! The more support structures you can put in place to help you through the time, the sooner you'll be able to see the forest instead of just the trees.

Make a survival plan

The first few weeks with a newborn can be all about survival. Feed, burp, nappy, rock, soothe, and then the baby naps; you try to get a few frantic bites of food into you (or take a shower – miraculous!) and then the baby's up again, and it's time to repeat the entire cycle. Simple, basic tasks like preparing meals, doing the laundry or going grocery shopping can suddenly seem monumental and completely overwhelming with a newborn who is not on any schedule yet. It's amazing how much time caring for a baby can take up! It might help to remind yourself that the only task which is truly important in these first few weeks is taking care of your newborn – that's your new job. Dishes and laundry can always wait, but learning how to soothe, comfort and care for your baby is necessary work which must be done right now.

Any work or preparation that you can do before you give birth will make a huge difference afterwards. Prepare as many meals as you can beforehand and store them in your freezer – simple, no-fuss meals which don't require a lot of preparation, such as lasagne or pasta or stews or soups you can just toss into a pot to warm up. Ask all of your friends and family members to bring a meal with them when they come to visit you. Consider ordering online meals for the first few weeks after the delivery; some websites even let others order meals for you.

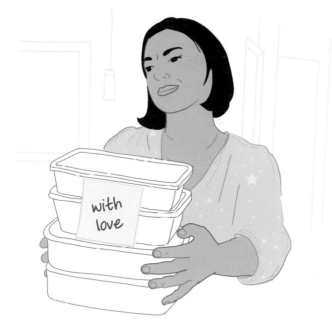

Let the guests do the work

You will have plenty of visitors in the first few weeks, and everyone is very eager to help out. Make sure you take real, practical advantage of their offers. If someone asks if they can bring you something, say 'yes!' and request a meal or extra nappies. And when visitors do come, keep the visits very short – neither you or your baby have a very long attention span at this point, and it's very easy to over-stimulate the baby or overextend yourself, especially when you're already so exhausted.

Lower your standards and the pressure you might otherwise put on yourself; there's no need to present a perfectly clean house or to worry about providing food or drinks for the many well-wishers who will stop by. Don't play the host – let them care for you, instead of the other way around. Sometimes wearing your pyjamas can help make this message very clear; if they don't take the hint and begin to overstay their welcome, ask your partner or a friend to gently move them towards the door.

Everyone's telling me what to do!

You'll probably find yourself receiving plenty of unsolicited parenting tips from family, friends and even complete strangers. While this can be incredibly frustrating, and can also undermine your fragile confidence in your own parenting skills, try not to take it to heart. Remember that most advice is well-intentioned, and use the following methods to try to deflect unhelpful comments:

- Rather than becoming defensive, let a comment wash off of you with a mild, self-deprecating response: 'Maybe he does look overdressed, but that's the look I'm going for – puffy snowman'.
- Sometimes honesty is the best policy; it's okay to say that a comment hurts your feelings, or to ask someone to refrain from offering advice.
- If it's a family member, tell them you appreciate their input, and you'll be sure to ask for their advice and help in the days and weeks to come; this helps put the emphasis on advice you've asked for, rather than advice you didn't.

Professional helpers

It helps tremendously to have some professional help, if you can afford it. A postnatal doula is someone skilled in breastfeeding, newborn care and household organization. She can sweep into your house for an afternoon, clean up the mess, prepare a meal, help with any breastfeeding difficulties, and teach you newborn skills. You can also hire a night nurse for the first few weeks; someone who can take care of the baby during the night while you catch up on some valuable sleep. Even if you're breastfeeding exclusively, you could wake up to feed the baby and hand the baby over afterwards so that the night attendant can burp, change and rock the baby while you go back to bed. If you can afford to have a cleaner for a while, hire one – that's one less job for you to do. If these services are cost-prohibitive, consider asking close friends or relatives if they can help out with tasks like cleaning or laundry.

> Mum brought round food for a week, kissed and left. Never loved her more. #tiredandsore

Team up with your partner

Most couples will find themselves fighting more after the arrival of a new baby than at any other point in their relationship, and research has shown that this arises from questions about money, work, the division of labour, and status within the relationship. Weathering and resolving the arguments in a way that makes both parties happy is difficult. Try to keep your sense of humour – laugh at your frazzled new life, rather than taking it too seriously. It's also a good idea to acknowledge what you've both lost – your life with just the two of you, your spontaneity (only temporarily) and your ability to pursue your own interests without interruption. And no matter what, don't try to keep score: both of you are exhausted, both of you are making huge sacrifices, both of you are finding this difficult. It's impossible to split all of the work 50/50, so appreciate your partner's help and effort with love and kindness.

Condensed idea
Support and a sense of humour will help you weather the transition from person to parent

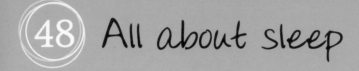

All about sleep

The first few weeks and months are hard. Your sleep is constantly broken and interrupted by a baby who's on a different schedule. While the entire world can start to look pretty hazy during this time, it helps to remember that this is a phase, and like all phases, it will pass.

Surviving the night

An adult has a 90-minute sleep cycle, but a baby's is only 60 minutes long. Which means that the baby can take a one-hour nap and wake up feeling refreshed, while you will be woken in the deepest part of your sleep-cycle, and waking up will feel a bit like you're clawing your way to consciousness through layers of cement. Unfortunately, in the first few months, it's normal for a baby to wake up for a feeding every two hours (their tiny stomachs don't hold much food, so they need small, frequent snacks).

Taking shifts with your partner may allow each of you to get the benefit of at least one completed sleep cycle, although this is much harder for the breastfeeding woman. If it's possible to pump and store breast milk for at least one feed during the night, your partner can give the baby this feed while you sleep straight through until the next feed, at which point your partner can sleep while you get up. If pumping is not yet an option, you can wake up just long enough to feed the baby then hand him over to your partner to burp, change the nappy and sooth him back to sleep. Keeping the baby very close to the bed makes night-time feeds much easier. Childbirth educator and author Penny Simkin recommends calculating how many hours you normally sleep during the night, and then staying in bed until you've had those hours. This means that even though you're waking up for feeds and baby care, you're going right back to bed again as soon as those tasks are done, and aren't actually starting your day until you've had your 6 or 8 hours, even if this means staying in bed from 10 p.m. until noon the following day.

Night-time tips

While each baby is different, you can start to use these tricks between two to four months to help get your little one to sleep for a bit longer at night:

- Lose the dummy. If your baby learns to sleep with a dummy in his mouth, he'll keep waking up when it falls out, and will expect you to put it back in for him every time. By 3–4 months, he's able to use self-soothing techniques like thumb sucking, which means he'll learn to comfort himself in the night rather than waking up and expecting it from you.
- Babies who go to sleep earlier sleep for longer. This helps prevent your baby from getting over-tired, at which point adrenaline kicks in and actually makes falling asleep harder rather than easier.
- Give your baby up to 10 minutes to try to figure out how to fall asleep on his own. Yes, he'll cry during this time, but if he learns to fall asleep on his own even once, it's an incredibly valuable lesson, and one that he may be able to repeat in the future. (Never do this with a newborn.)
- When you go in to comfort your baby, do as little as possible to soothe him – try patting, singing, talking and stroking rather than picking him up.

Safe sleep

We still don't fully understand what causes Sudden Infant Death Syndrome (SIDS), but we know that the highest risk is during the first six months. Smoking during the pregnancy, living in a household with a smoker, or placing your baby in a face-down position to sleep have all been associated with increased risk of SIDS, and formula-fed infants have double the risk of dying from SIDS than their breast-fed counterparts.

In order to help prevent SIDS, it's important that the baby sleeps on a firm mattress without extra pillows or blankets around, as these can get trapped around the baby's face and increase the chance of suffocation. Using a sleep sack (a wearable blanket which fastens around the baby) helps avoid this, as does keeping the bassinet or crib free of bumpers, stuffed animals, soft bedding or other props. It's also important to ensure the room is well ventilated, keep the overall room temperature cool (around 20°C (68°F), and avoid over-bundling your baby in too many layers (including hats). Make sure the mattress cover is tight-fitting, there are no gaps between the mattress and the crib, and that you're using a crib or bassinet made after 2000, when safety standards changed. And of course, place your baby on his back to sleep!

> I'm going to let new dad do the midnight feed tonight. He's excited but I'm over the moon! #zzzzzzzz

Sleep routines

For the first two months of life, it's impossible to establish a routine. Your baby may even have 'day-night reversal', meaning he'll be more wakeful at night than during the day for the first few weeks. Exposing your baby to sunlight during the day and keeping lights low and noises soft at night may help reverse this pattern more quickly. Do whatever you can to keep your baby asleep for as long as possible (the most you

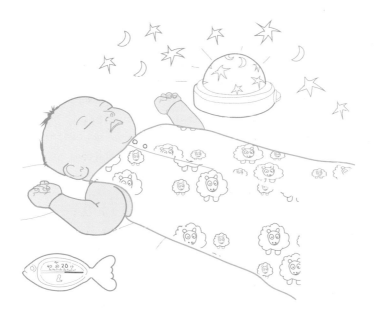

can expect is about four hours of continuous sleep): swaddle him, rock him, encourage sucking (either nursing, or using a thumb or pacifier), go for walks or car-rides, and sing or make a shushing noise. During this time it's impossible to spoil your baby or set up bad sleep habits.

After four months, the baby becomes more aware of his environment, which means routine becomes more important. Work on teaching your baby to fall asleep on his own by no longer letting him fall asleep on you, or while feeding. Put him down when he's drowsy rather than fast asleep. Creating a bedtime routine (bath, feed, lullaby, bed) and doing this every night helps mark bedtime. It's important to keep sleep times and locations consistent as well.

condensed idea
There's no such thing as the perfect mum who never sleeps and still looks after her baby well

(49) Baby blues

Many women experience the baby blues, which is thought to be due to the huge hormonal, emotional and physical changes that happen rapidly after the birth. They are usually short lived, but can sometimes lead to a serious depression which needs to be recognized and treated.

Why do I feel sad?

You've just had a baby, you're really happy about this, so why do you keep crying all the time? While this may seem incredibly incongruous, the baby blues is a well-documented phenomenon that affects around 80 per cent of all women; it starts a few days to a week after delivery and lasts for up to two weeks. While the exact cause of the baby blues is not fully understood, it's probably a potent combination of hormonal fluctuations (the loss of the high levels of feel-good oestrogen, in particular), sleep deprivation and exhaustion, emotional changes and sometimes physical pain. It's common for many women to feel sad, tearful, overwhelmed, guilty, isolated, resentful and anxious in the first few days after the birth. Even though this is normal and expected (at least by healthcare professionals), many women are surprised by how moody, unpredictable and emotional they become.

The good news about the baby blues is that they usually only last for a few weeks at most. Being able to acknowledge and express your feelings, particularly the negative ones as well as the positive, definitely helps, as does nurturing and support from your partner, family members and friends. Experiencing the baby blues is not necessarily a predictor for long-term depression, but if you find that the symptoms persist beyond two weeks, it's definitely time to talk with your doctor about it.

Varying degrees of depression

Postnatal depression (PND) is the umbrella term used to describe a large spectrum of mood disorders affecting new mothers within the first year of the birth of their baby. These disorders include postnatal depression, postnatal anxiety, postnatal obsessive compulsive disorder and postnatal psychosis; the baby blues also fall under this umbrella, at the mildest end of the spectrum. While it's difficult to tell exactly how many women experience these disorders, as they're frequently unrecognized, misdiagnosed or ignored, it's thought that 10–20 per cent of all mothers develop a more serious postnatal mood disorder.

Many of the symptoms of postnatal depression are vague and hard to pinpoint, but in general they include feelings of loss, hopelessness and sadness, fatigue and lack of energy, insomnia, lack of appetite, inability to laugh, concentrate or enjoy pre-baby activities, frequent crying, irritability, detachment and, in severe cases, thoughts of harming yourself and your baby. In cases of postnatal anxiety or postnatal obsessive compulsive disorder, symptoms

> Decided to stop feeling guilty about feeling sad and phoned BFF. Good friends are a life-saver. #goodenoughmum

also include sudden panic attacks or a racing heart, obsessive negative thoughts, preoccupation with cleanliness and germs, doubts about your ability to care for the baby, excessively elaborate routines to complete simple activities, fear of leaving the house, impulses to run away and hide, inability to comprehend what you're reading, shaking or trembling, fear of being alone with the baby, or recurring thoughts or daydreams of doing harm to the baby or yourself (or outside harm occurring to the baby).

If you or your family have a history of depression, you're at greater risk of developing a mood disorder. Other risks include stressful life events coinciding with the birth, such as a job loss, death of a loved one or marital conflict. Lack of support, an unwanted pregnancy or having a baby with a difficult temperament can also trigger a latent depression.

Good mothers get depressed too

With postnatal depression, it's very easy to feel as if you're all alone and that something is wrong with you. Many women find themselves reluctant to admit their feelings to themselves, and associate the depression with a personality failure on their part. In all cases, the sooner the condition is recognized and treatment can begin, the shorter the length and severity of the disorder. In some cases, putting extra support structures in place, or receiving counselling or therapy, are enough to turn the situation around. Attending a postnatal support group and meeting with other women who may be feeling similar can be hugely helpful. Talking about your feelings and having them acknowledged in a caring, non-judgmental environment is one of the best ways to heal. In other cases, a short course of antidepressants can make a huge difference.

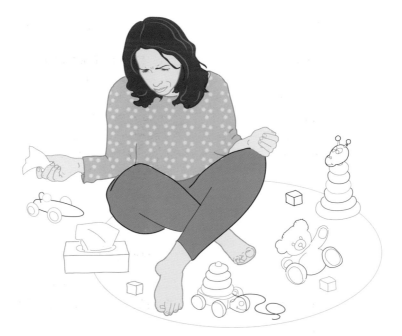

Places to get help

Increasing media coverage and public awareness during the last decade means that the stigma formerly associated with postnatal depression is fading away. These days there are many excellent resources available for postnatal depression, including many online ones, which are based in certain countries but can be accessed from anywhere.

- UK: Postnatal Depression UK (www.pni.org.uk) and Home Start, a charity focused on pairing volunteers with vulnerable mothers (www.home-start.org.uk).
- USA: www.postpartumsupport.net and www.ppdsupportpage. com; US National PPD hotline: 1-800-PPD-MOMS.
- Australia: Post and Antenatal Depression Association (www. panda.org.au).
- Canada: Pacific Post Partum Support Society (www.postpartum. org); www.postpartumprogress.com
- Books: *Down Came the Rain* by Brooke Shields; *The Pregnancy and Postpartum Anxiety Workbook* by Gyoekoe, Wiegartz and Miller; *Mothering the New Mother* by Sally Placksin.
- Thousands of other local and online resources are available: speak with your midwife, doctor, health visitor or social worker to find out about local support groups and assistance.

condensed idea
Eat well, rest more, talk honestly and the baby blues will subside a little bit sooner

A new identity

Parenthood is a lifelong transition, an evolution that will teach you and change you profoundly for the rest of your life. You will be faced with endless daily decisions, which will push your boundaries and lead to inevitable (and forgivable) mistakes.

Give yourself time

Parenthood is an incredibly intimidating task – accepting full responsibility for meeting the needs of another person, and then teaching, moulding and shaping that little person into a decent human being and functioning member of society. The good news is: you don't have to know all of that straightaway! You learn how to be a parent as you go along. Your first lessons are very simple; rocking, feeding, soothing and burping require a lot of time and physical care, but at least you're not having to teach the difference between right and wrong yet, or how to be a moral person in an immoral world – thankfully, those lessons come later, once you're ready for them.

You could spend years gearing up for parenthood, reading every parenting book on the market, debating the merits of a parent-centred approach (creating scheduled feedings, sleep training and so on) versus a child-centred approach (feeding on demand, co-sleeping, attachment parenting), and learning about the latest research and trends. However, your best parenting will come when you let all of that go and just dive in. You already have all of the tools, knowledge and resources you need to be a good parent inside you, without any extra reading or learning required. Parenting will scare you, confuse you and keep you up at night, but the best way to learn to parent is to just do it. Only then will

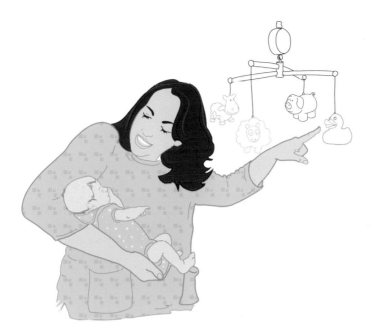

you discover what's on the other side of that sleepless night, that scary moment or that confusion, and you can bet it will be followed by greater understanding and confidence.

Follow your child

It's impossible to be a perfect parent. Don't even try! Accept from the very beginning that you will make mistakes (lots of them) and that this is totally okay. Every mistake you make is an opportunity to learn. Luckily, your child isn't looking for perfection; she's looking for your love and engagement. The greatest gift you can give to your child is your presence. Be present in her world. Pay attention to the things she's paying attention to (in the beginning, this is as simple as noticing what she's looking at and naming it for her) and listen to what she's telling you (you'll be amazed by how much she can communicate with you non-verbally in the beginning, and then later with her new and magical words). Put down your smartphone and all of the trappings of modern society and give her some of your undivided attention and time.

Every child is different – and that is what is so special about them. No child will develop at the same rate as another, or learn in the same way, or have the same thoughts or preferences or personality. You can use books as a reference, or follow the guidelines of experts, but the best authority on your child is your child. And the more you sit back and observe what your child is up to, the more you will learn and understand who she is. It's incredibly easy for us to impose our own pre-conceived notions onto a child, but if you're patient and actually watch rather than assume, you will be surprised, every time.

Trust your instincts

Your child is brand new, without any of the learned behaviours of modern society or intellectual reasoning. She's fresh and curious, with no assumptions about the world or about other people. As scary as it might seem at first, she will look to you to teach her about the world.

You know you're a mother when...

- You find yourself swaying and rocking when you don't even have your baby in your arms.
- You discover some kind of dried something on your top (sick? milk? who knows?) which you hadn't even noticed before, and you just shrug.
- You know all of the words to at least three lullabies.
- You clean a dummy with your mouth.
- You finally know that you will get everything that you need to do done – just more slowly, and on your baby's schedule.
- You say at least once a day, 'I'm not cut out for this', but in your heart know that you wouldn't trade it for the world.

She might not understand why she's cold and wet or hungry, but she will instinctively seek you out as the person who can figure it out for her. And gradually, as you observe and get to know your baby, you'll get much better and faster at understanding what she wants and then providing it for her. Trust your instincts. You already know more about your baby than anyone else in the world – after all, she's lived

> I can't imagine my baby talking or going to school, but I know it will happen. Hope I can give her everything she'll need. Love her so. #proudmum

inside you, beneath your heart, for nine months already. Trust the inner voice in your head, or that feeling in your gut. Much of what we learn from our children can't be put into words, but we just know, sometimes, without being able to explain it. Trust that feeling, and listen to your heart.

Trusting your instincts also means trusting your child. Many of us want to sweep in and do everything for our children, in our quest to provide them with every tool, every resource, every experience and every success. The harder thing to do is to trust that our children are more than capable of figuring things out for themselves, without our constant help. Trust that she will learn to sit up on her own, when she's ready, and that she'll learn to use the toilet in her own time. As your child gets older, there will be plenty of lessons she'll only be able to learn if you withdraw slightly, so that she can fall down and learn to pick herself back up. It's very scary to let her fail at something, but trust that she will figure it out, and remember that the bigger gift you are giving her is trust in herself and her own abilities. That's your real job as a parent.

Condensed idea
You and your baby are the best parenting authorities out there

Glossary

Antenatal Before birth; prenatal.

Apgar score The score of a test given one minute and five minutes after birth to assess the baby's skin colour, pulse, reflexes, muscle tone and breathing. A perfect score is 10.

Baby blues Mild depression that develops a few days after giving birth.

Biophysical profile (BPP) An ultrasound test to check foetal breathing, movement and tone, and the volume of amniotic fluid.

Birth plan A parents' list of their preferences for birth management, including preferences for pain relief, induction and so on.

Braxton Hicks contractions 'Practice' contractions that begin around six weeks before birth.

Breech presentation An unusual position of the baby in the uterus, where the baby's bottom or feet face the mother's cervix.

Cerclage A type of stitch performed on a weak or incompetent cervix to keep it closed and prevent a premature birth.

Cervical ripening A process that occurs during early labour, making the cervix soft and thin.

Cervix The narrow, lower end of the uterus that thins and opens during labour.

Caesarean section A surgical procedure in which incisions are made in the abdomen and uterus to deliver a baby. Also called a C-section.

Chorionic villus sampling (CVS) A diagnostic test using placental tissues to screen for genetic abnormalities such as Down's syndrome.

Colostrum A nutrient-rich, sticky yellow fluid secreted by the breasts for the first few days after birth.

Contraction A contraction of the uterine muscle, which tightens the uterus and dilates the cervix.

Crowning The moment during labour when the baby's head can be seen at the vaginal opening.

C-section See caesarean section.

Doula Childbirth assistant who is specially trained to assist mothers during labour and liaise with medical staff.

Down's syndrome A congenital disorder caused by an extra chromosome.

Eclampsia A condition resulting from untreated pre-eclampsia characterized by seizures, very high blood pressure and abnormal blood tests.

Ectopic pregnancy A pregnancy where the fertilized egg has implanted outside the uterus, usually in a Fallopian tube.

Effacement The thinning and softening of the cervix during labour.

Epidural A type of anaesthesia administered into the base of the spine constantly, via a catheter, to numb the lower body.

Episiotomy A surgical incision in the perineum performed to enlarge the vaginal opening during delivery.

Foetal monitoring The monitoring of a baby's heartbeat during labour.

Foetal movement counts A test where women of 27+ weeks gestation count how often their baby moves within an hour.

Foetus The medical name for a baby from 8 weeks of pregnancy until birth.

Fontanelles Soft spots on a baby's head that allow the bony plates of its skull to flex during birth.

Forceps Surgical 'tongs' that are used to help deliver a baby.

Full-term A baby born at 37–42 weeks' gestation.

Genetic screening Tests performed during pregnancy to detect genetic abnormalities such as Down's syndrome or Trisomy 18 (Edward's syndrome) in the foetus.

Gestation Generally counted in weeks, the period of time a baby has been carried in the uterus (gestation is counted from the first day of the last menstrual period).

Gynaecologist (GYN) A doctor specializing in women's reproductive health.

Incompetent cervix The term for a cervix that opens before labour begins.

Induction The use of medical drugs to encourage labour to begin.

Labour The process of childbirth, from early contractions to the delivery of the baby and later the placenta.

Lactation The production of milk in the breasts that follows from childbirth.

Lamaze A method of controlling pain during childbirth through relaxation and rhythmic breathing patterns.

Lanugo The fine, downy hair that temporarily covers a foetus from 26 weeks or so until birth.

Latching on The movement in which the baby makes the correct connection to the nipple in order to breastfeed.

Linea nigra A dark, vertical line that develops on the abdomen during pregnancy.

Lochia A form of vaginal discharge and bleeding that begins after delivery and tapers off gradually over around six weeks.

Meconium The baby's greenish-brown first stool.

Moulding The temporary reshaping of a baby's head during birth, which occurs due to pressure from the birth canal and pelvic bones.

Neonatal The time from a baby's birth to 28 days after the birth.

Neural tube defect A birth defect that affects the baby's brain or spine.

Obstetrician A doctor specializing in pregnancy, labour and the postnatal period.

Oxytocin A hormone secreted by the body during birth that causes uterine contractions.

Paediatrician A doctor specializing in the medical care of infants and children.

Perinatal The time immediately before and after birth.

Perineum The area on a woman's body between the vagina and rectum.

Placenta An organ that develops in the uterus to connect the foetus to the woman's body via the umbilical cord.

Postnatal period The time period between delivery and 6–8 weeks after the birth.

Pre-eclampsia A medical condition during pregnancy characterized by high blood pressure and blood proteins; if untreated, can progress to eclampsia.

Premature baby A baby born before 37 weeks' gestation.

Premature labour Labour that occurs between 20 and 37 weeks' gestation.

Prenatal Before birth.

Show The passing of the mucus plug that sealed the cervical canal during pregnancy.

Spinal block A type of anaesthesia administered into the base of the spine once, via injection, to numb the lower body.

TENS (transcutaneous electrical nerve stimulation) A hand-held device that delivers mild bursts of electricity through the skin, which works to alleviate pain.

Transitional labour The end of the first stage of labour when the cervix dilates through strong, very fast recurring contractions.

Trimester A time period of three months; pregnancy is divided into three trimesters.

Umbilical cord A cord of tissue that connects the foetus to the placenta.

Uterus A hollow, muscular organ in which the foetus grows.

Vernix A white, creamy substance that covers the foetus during the last trimester.

Index

Acknowledgements

Author acknowledgements

This book owes a tremendous debt to the following: Sarah Tomley, for her editorial skills and endless encouragement, Tracy Killick for seeing the potential and getting the job done, Emily Milcarek, who would have never let me *not* write this book, Debbie Paley for helping to mould me into the midwife I am today, Stacey Rees for your trust, Amy Reiter Stoutimore for being the best reader a girl could have, James for your everything, every day, and Ethan, my greatest teacher.

Picture credits

Incidental images used throughout.
Fotolia: Anna; Arôme; Willee Cole; Draganm; Elinor33; Erica Guilane-Nachez; Ilyaka; Leremy; Mayboro; Milanpetrovic; Adrian Niederhäuser; Zoran Popovic; Tpandd
Shutterstock: Potapov Alexander; Docent; W. Jarva; Osijan
istockphoto: Bubaone

Quercus Publishing Plc
55 Baker Street, 7th Floor,
South Block, London W1U 8EW

First published in 2013

A catalogue record of this book is available from the British Library

ISBN 978 1 78206 132 8

Printed and bound in China

10 9 8 7 6 5 4 3 2 1

Produced for Quercus Publishing Plc by Tracy Killick Art Direction and Design

Commissioning editor: Sarah Tomley (of www.editorsonline.org)
Designer: Tracy Killick
Project editor: Alice Bowden
Proof reader: Louise Abbott
Illustrator: Victoria Woodgate (www.vickywoodgate.com)
Indexer: Hilary Bird